Perspectives on Rehabilitation and Dementia

of related interest

Dementia and Social Inclusion
Marginalised groups and marginalised areas of dementia research,
care and practice
Edited by Anthea Innes, Carole Archibald and Charlie Murphy
ISBN 1 84310 174 2

Including the Person with Dementia in Designing
and Delivering Care
'I Need to Be Me!'
Elizabeth Barnett
ISBN 1 85302 740 5

Explorations in Dementia
Theoretical and Research Studies into the Experience of Remediable and
Enduring Cognitive Losses
Michael Bender
ISBN 1 84310 040 1

Understanding Dementia
The Man with the Worried Eyes
Richard Cheston and Michael Bender
ISBN 1 85302 479 1

The Perspectives of People with Dementia
Research Methods and Motivations
Edited by Heather Wilkinson
ISBN 1 84310 001 0

Integrating Care for Older People
New Care for Old – A Systems Approach
Christopher Foote and Christine Stanners
ISBN 1 84310 010 X

Care Services for Later Life
Transformations and Critiques
Edited by Tony Warnes, Mike Nolan and Lorna Warren
ISBN 1 85302 852 5

Healing Arts Therapies and Person-Centred Dementia Care
Edited by Anthea Innes and Karen Hatfield
ISBN 1 84310 038 X
Bradford Dementia Group Good Practice Guides

Hearing the Voice of People with Dementia
Opportunities and Obstacles
Malcolm Goldsmith
ISBN 1 85302 406 6

Perspectives on Rehabilitation and Dementia

Edited by Mary Marshall

Jessica Kingsley Publishers
London and Philadelphia

First published in 2005
by Jessica Kingsley Publishers
116 Pentonville Road
London N1 9JB, UK
and
400 Market Street, Suite 400
Philadelphia, PA 19106, USA

www.jkp.com

Copyright © Jessica Kingsley Publishers 2005

Library of Congress Cataloging in Publication Data

Perspectives on rehabilitation and dementia / Edited by Mary Marshall.
    p. cm.
Includes bibliographical references and index.
ISBN 1-84310-286-2 (pbk.)
1. Dementia--Patients--Rehabilitation. I. Marshall, Mary.
RC521.P427 2004
616.8'3--dc22

                                            2004010447

British Library Cataloguing in Publication Data
A CIP catalogue record for this book is available from the British Library

ISBN-13 978 1 84310 286 1
ISBN-10 1 84310 286 2

Printed and Bound in Great Britain by
Athenaeum Press, Gateshead, Tyne and Wear

Contents

Part Three: Specific Professional Perspectives

Part Four: Specific Settings

Part Five: Specific Interventions

Part Six: Specific Difficulties

Part Seven: Conclusion

List of Tables

List of Figures

Preface

This book grew out of a conference on rehabilitation and dementia hosted by the King's Fund in December 2001. It was clear, at the time, that people with dementia were missing out on the increasing resources available for rehabilitation and intermediate care. Participants were very appreciative of the input on the day and there was an obvious need for a book. This is not the book which would have resulted if it had been produced immediately after the conference. The time that was available has meant that it is both broader and deeper.

This book was made possible by a grant from the Scottish Executive to whom warm thanks are due. They were willing to support what they perceived as a useful contribution to dementia care.

Thanks are also due to all the contributors who provided chapters based on hard-won experience. It is hoped that their willingness to share this will improve the lives and opportunities of people with dementia and their carers.

Mary Marshall

PART ONE

Perspectives on the Field as a Whole

CHAPTER 1

Perspectives on Rehabilitation and Dementia

Mary Marshall

'Rehabilitation' and 'dementia' are not words that have been associated to any great extent until recently. This is partly because they were not felt to be compatible and partly because they are both complex terms and need to be very carefully and thoughtfully connected. This book is an attempt to show the usefulness of linking the two words in a way that clarifies them for both theory and practice. Numerous experts have contributed their thinking in short papers. This opening chapter attempts to provide some structure for approaching the range of perspectives, and to raise some issues which will be revisited and reviewed in the closing chapter.

The reasons for this book

First we need to consider why there is increasing interest in rehabilitation at this point in the development of work with people with dementia. Much of the most useful thinking about dementia has happened as a result of applying thinking from other fields and reflecting on the extent to which such concepts illuminate dementia care. Thus we borrowed 'challenging behaviour' from learning disability and found a good fit. We borrowed 'person-centred' from social psychology and found a profound challenge to existing approaches. Some theorists are looking at child development and finding helpful models from Piaget.

One of the pressures in dementia care is to make it respectable, in the sense of making it mainstream, in the hope that people with dementia will cease to be marginalized. If we can label some of dementia care 'rehabilitation', we stand some chance of mainstream healthcare both understanding and taking an interest in it. The real excitement, enthusiasm and resources of health services are for conditions where there is some treatment. Traditionally, dementia care was always downgraded because there was 'no treatment for it'. Cholinesterase inhibitors have significantly raised the level of interest in dementia by providing a treatment. However, these are not a cure and they only work in about a quarter of people with Alzheimer's disease. If we can make a case for rehabilitation and dementia, then perhaps we can generate a real interest and excitement: this is a term with wide currency in mainstream health. As such, it might help the mainstream to understand what we in dementia care are trying to achieve.

But is the use of the term more than this? Can it help us to develop our thinking and understanding of dementia care itself? This book will need to answer this question. Although there is value in better communication with mainstream healthcare, our major concern must always be to improve our thinking and practice.

One of the problems we have in dementia care is use of terms like person-centred care and holistic care, which have a motherhood and apple-pie feel about them and mean little to those outside our field (and indeed to the majority of those in our field who have not really been exposed to the latest thinking). There have been many valiant attempts to apply these approaches and some hard thinking about the difficulties of doing this (for example Packer 2000). Perhaps the use of well-established concepts like rehabilitation will influence a wider audience.

One of the reasons this matter is so topical is a rather belated realization that many older people 'blocking beds' are people with dementia who have on the whole missed out on rehabilitation for a range of complex reasons to do with expertise and expectations. This book will need to clarify how this has happened and what should be done about it. Delayed discharge, as it is now referred to, is a matter of great concern to health policy in all four nations of the UK, so there is a plethora of policies. We need to turn our attention to the extent to which these policies help people with dementia as well as looking at the actual practice of key professional groups, especially the Allied Health Professionals (AHPs) and nurses.

Another reason why this topic is 'hot' at the moment is the maturing of dementia care itself. We now have a richness of approaches and experience which allows us to reflect and to make attempts to pull it together. It also allows us to interface with other fields, such as palliative care, to see how we can improve our practice all the way along the journey that dementia itself takes individuals and their families.

It is customary in books about dementia to assert that it is the increasing numbers of people with dementia which has raised the levels of interest in it. This must in part be the case, but equally important has been the realization that this is a fascinating area of work, which challenges our imaginations, our intellects and our practice development in very fundamental ways. This book has to contribute to this as one of its objectives. Its other objectives are a bit more straightforward:

- To sensitize professionals, planners, managers and commissioners to the potential of rehabilitation with people with dementia.
- To give examples.
- To provide guidance on extending work practice.
- To guide readers to further reading.

What do we mean by rehabilitation?

There are numerous definitions of rehabilitation. The common thread between them is the positive approach. People can function better with help. Clearly, people with dementia are rarely going to return to their level of functioning before they had dementia, but many can function a great deal better than they do at present.

This book looks at four approaches to rehabilitation and dementia:

1. Rehabilitation after some acute physical episode such as an acute infection, surgery or treatment to the heart or lungs. This is the most familiar use of the word and most easily understood, this generally happens in an acute ward or some other place designated especially for rehabilitation. It is usually undertaken by nurses and AHPs.

2. Rehabilitation after an acute episode of challenging behaviour. These episodes often require an admission so that drug regimes can be reviewed and other interventions considered. Sometimes it is about getting to the root of the problem and sorting out the factors exacerbating the behaviour. Sometimes the behaviour is considered to be due to brain damage alone and decisions must then made about the best place for the person to stay until this phase of the condition passes.

3. Cognitive rehabilitation is increasingly recognized as possible and important and there is increasing evidence as well as practice base. The aim is to make use of aspects of the brain which still function, rather than assuming an inevitable decline for which nothing can be done.

4. Rehabilitation can be seen as a general approach to working with people with dementia in that it stresses the need for proactive and positive interactions. The assumption is that most people can function better if they receive appropriate help.

There are some key concepts in all approaches to rehabilitation, which should have equal applicability when working with people with dementia; this book needs to address how they are best achieved if there is to be real usefulness in the concept of rehabilitation and dementia.

Teamwork

All texts on rehabilitation stress that it is not the prerogative of one profession. It needs to be a shared approach between all those working with people with dementia, all of whom will have a role but none optimally effective on their own.

Working with families and other support mechanisms

Very few people with dementia can manage entirely on their own; none of us can. We are all part of couples, families and friendship groups. Rehabilitation will be undermined if key people are not involved and will usually be enhanced if it is a shared endeavour.

Prostheses

Rehabilitation usually includes some aids, adaptations, tools or environmental modifications of some sort to make life easier for the person. This is a potentially very subtle concept when working with people with any kind of mental illness since prosthetics may be people as well as more tangible things.

Removing causes of excess (or unnecessary) disability

It is obviously sensible to address factors in the lives of people with dementia which prevent them from functioning as well as they can. These can occur at many levels and can include the impact of negative interactions on self-esteem and confidence as well as unhelpful environments, under-nutrition, untreated illness both medical and psychiatric, stress and so on. The diagram below provides a simple graphic to illustrate this point. The brain damage is a given; everything else can be 'treated', both factors which are positive in their impact and factors which are negative. This book addresses a number of them.

Learning and motivation

Rehabilitation is assumed to require these two qualities to be successful. Clearly both are difficult for someone with dementia, who may have impaired learning and insufficient understanding to be motivated. The contributors to this book explain how rehabilitation is possible in these circumstances.

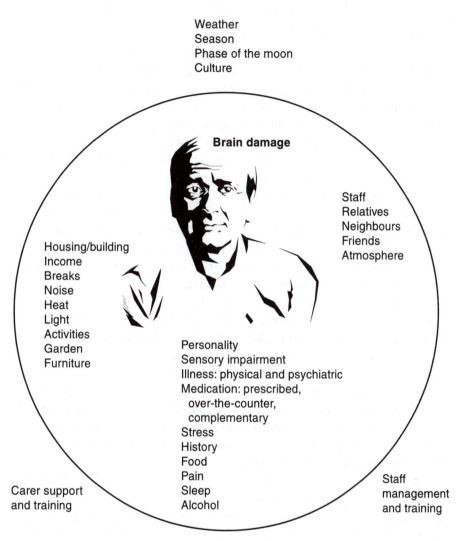

Weather
Season
Phase of the moon
Culture

Brain damage

Staff
Relatives
Neighbours
Friends
Atmosphere

Housing/building
Income
Breaks
Noise
Heat
Light
Activities
Garden
Furniture

Personality
Sensory impairment
Illness: physical and psychiatric
Medication: prescribed,
  over-the-counter,
  complementary
Stress
History
Food
Pain
Sleep
Alcohol

Carer support
and training

Staff
management
and training

Figure 1.1 Factors which can cause unnecessary disability

A focus

Rehabilitation cannot sort out every aspect of people's lives. What is the appropriate focus for rehabilitation of people with dementia? Is it well-being generally or specific problems? The answer will clearly be complicated by the fact that this is a progressive condition.

What do we mean by dementia?

The next word which needs attention is 'dementia' itself. This term is most usefully thought of as having at least three sides, although no object has three faces so a better metaphor might be a tetrahedron (i.e. with four sides). One of them should be the individual who is experiencing the condition in their own unique way. Everybody has a different pathway through this disease.

One side of the tetrahedron is the *medical approach*, which stresses the brain damage itself. Doctors and others who emphasize this view tend to attribute most of what we see and what the person experiences to the extent and location of brain damage. This can be a rather negative approach given that there is little we can do about brain damage, although research into preventing the disease itself is gaining momentum (Gow and Gilhooly 2003). People who see dementia primarily in terms of brain damage tend to suggest that the main focus of effort should be on the people who support humane and compassionate care. This approach assumes that doctors are the experts in dementia.

Another side of the tetrahedron is the *social or disability approach* best illustrated by Figure 1.1. The approach suggests that a lot of the experience of dementia depends on the person, their background and health, and on all the factors in their environment. Much recent work has focused on the interactions between the relative or helper and the person with dementia (Kitwood 1997), and perhaps too little on groups of people and the way they interact. This is changing rapidly as groups of people with dementia are seen as beneficial and researchers are focusing their attention on relationships and friendships between people with dementia. This approach assumes that all professions, relatives and friends have useful things to say about dementia.

A third side of the tetrahedron is the *citizenship model*, which suggests that people with dementia have a unique contribution to make to our society and the extent of this can be facilitated. Many people with dementia go through a period of great creativity if they are given the opportunity to express it. Other contributions such as emotional veracity and humour, as well as an example of fortitude in the face of major trauma, are often undervalued. This approach assumes that people with dementia are the experts on dementia, although we may have to improve our communication skills to understand what they are saying.

This book is based on this four-sided approach to dementia to give a true and rounded view. Clearly, different authors have different backgrounds and emphasis but all contribute to our understanding of how rehabilitation and this multidimensional view of dementia go together.

Perspectives

The contributions to this book are all experts in dementia care and include some people with dementia. They are people with enormously rich experience and many of them have been very influential in current thinking about dementia and dementia care. Others are working at the coalface and this is their first opportunity to share their approach. They were all asked to write about what rehabilitation meant for them. Although every effort was made to cover all the different approaches to dementia and the different professional perspectives, it was never going to be possible to cover all the ground. The result has, however, been chapters of extraordinary richness and diversity. For all the contributors the concept of rehabilitation proved highly relevant and applicable. This book is also intended to be a journey, so no attempt will be made here to influence the experience by presenting any sort of summary. The last chapter will attempt this. It will try and draw out the threads that link the contributions and the ways in which the concept of rehabilitation in all four uses of the term is illuminated in its application to the task of improving the lives of people with dementia and their carers.

The contributions have been arranged to start with general points and then move to specific perspectives. The exception to this is Chapter 2 by Professor Jolley, which is a perspective of a consultant in old age psychiatry. However, it is placed at the start because it contains basic information about dementia which may be useful for readers from other fields. Other general chapters include Chapter 5, a review of the literature by Gail Mountain, Chapter 3, a historical perspective by Suzanne Cahill and Avril Dooley, and Chapter 4, a policy perspective by Kate Read.

References

Gow, J. and Gilhooly, M. (2003) *Risk Factors for Dementia and Cognitive Decline.* Glasgow: NHS Health Scotland.

Kitwood, T. (1997) *Dementia Reconsidered: The Person Comes First.* Buckingham: Open University Press.

Packer, T. (2000) 'Does person-centred care exist?' *Journal of Dementia Care 10*, 3, 19–21.

CHAPTER 2

Why Do People with Dementia Become Disabled?

David Jolley

Introduction

At the time when pioneers were realizing the need to generate special services for older people with mental health problems in the UK of the late 1960s, the main identifiable provision was within long-stay wards of mental hospitals. These offered blocks of 50 beds per dormitory for aged individuals of one gender alongside a cavernous day room and limited toilet and bathing facilities. Nursing numbers were few, doctors' visits infrequent, brief and largely devoted to prescribing for inter-current physical illnesses or signing the death certificate (Jolley and Arie 1978; Whitehead 1978). In the official returns it was declared that no occupational therapy, physiotherapy nor clinical psychology staff were delegated to work on these wards. This was not seen to be a problem. It was assumed the residents would not benefit from such expertise.

In most hospitals patients were of mixed diagnoses, brought together simply by the availability of a bed, their age and the perceived chronicity and incurability of their condition. Most old people with dementia would die within twelve months of admission. None would survive two winters (Roth 1955). These were the people with dementia whose behaviour within the course of the condition had become such that they were deemed 'psychiatric'. Many others were being cared for at home, in the workhouse or its successor institutions or long-stay 'geriatric' wards. For then, as now, dementia was ubiquitous and hardly differentiated from the 'normal' consequences of great age: summed up as 'senility'. This was to be accepted and tolerated as an inevitable cost of longevity.

Margery Warren had demonstrated, within the chronic sick wards of West Middlesex, that active treatment and rehabilitation could transform the last years of people who had been set aside, warehoused in dependency to await death (Warren 1960). Peter Townsend and others had suggested that replacing work-house regimes and philosophy with domestic scale accommodation and more optimistic approaches would release suppressed vitality, activity and happiness amongst potential 'inmates' (Townsend 1962). So the time and the scene was ripe for revision of established views and practices.

There has been a revolution in the provision of services for the mentally ill in the UK and in many other parts of the world. The transformation of services for older people with dementia and other mental disorders has shown a lead which is being followed in the rest of the world. Nevertheless, most people with dementia spend most of their time alone or in the care of their family or non-specialist ser-vices unaware of their vulnerabilities and special needs. Specialist services may fall short of optimal performance in their totality or in parts because of lack of knowledge, limited vision or lack of resource (Arie and Jolley 1998).

Characteristics of dementia

Dementia is a relatively common condition, affecting roughly 5 per cent of people aged 65 years and beyond. It is age-related. Importantly a few individuals experience symptoms before the age of 60 years, symptoms are evident in 1 to 2 per cent of people in their 60s and 20 per cent or more of those in their 80s and beyond (Jorm, Korten and Henderson 1987). In most instances, its onset is insidious and its course progressive, though there are examples with sudden onset and progress by steps of deterioration, punctuating periods of 'plateau' impairment. It is debilitating and carries a reduced life expectation. Death may be preceded by a lengthy period of dependency, weight loss and inanition (Black and Jolley 1990).

'Dementia' is best looked on as a syndrome characterized as: 'an acquired global impairment of intellect, memory and personality, but without impairment of consciousness' (Lishman 1978). It may be caused by one or more of a number of underlying pathological processes, each with their particular features and prognosis. Alzheimer's disease is the most common of the dementing illnesses and responsible for most dementia encountered in practice. Vascular dementia, Lewy body dementia and fronto-temporal dementia are also relatively common illnesses with recognized pathology and neuropathology.

Dementia may occur as a symptom or consequence of other conditions including trauma to the brain, pressure on the brain or infections involving neurones or other intra-cranial structures. It may be consequent on malnutrition, especially lack of essential vitamins, or caused by toxicity from ingested com-pounds including alcohol, some medicines or elements, or because of failure of the kidney or liver to clear harmful metabolites. Inadequate circulation to the brain due to heart problems or reduced or raised blood pressure may induce acute or chronic 'brain failure', as may any condition reducing the oxygen concentration or increasing the carbon dioxide content within circulating blood. Hormonal problems including under or over activity of the thyroid gland, pituitary or adrenal glands, or diabetes in its various modes and complications, may result in neuronal damage and dementia. Other conditions, most notably depression and chronic intoxication with medicines, may mimic dementia but be reversible with appropriate treatment and leave no long-term sequelae.

Thus the common features of dementia, crossing the boundaries of particular diagnoses and aetiologies, are that it is:

- acquired: representing a change (deterioration) compared with previously established function
- global: involving all or most functions associated with intellect and memory, otherwise styled 'cognitive' functions, but also including 'personality'.

Personality is not easy to define and less easy to measure but represents the essence of a person. Change within its dimensions is malignant and contributes greatly to loss of ability and independence.

Cognitive losses

Impaired memory is the accepted hallmark symptom of dementia. Indeed a system of 'Memory Clinics' is now emerging, largely to encourage earlier presentation of people with dementia for assessment and consideration of treatment before damage has become firmly established (Lindesay et al. 2002).

Difficulties are most obviously evident with registering and retaining new information. Stories from long ago are retained, perhaps in a modified form, and may be rehearsed repeatedly. Habits and skills practised over decades may be even more securely programmed and remain available.

But the cognitive losses in dementia are not limited to dysmnesia; 'grasp' or comprehension of situations, understanding of questions, discussion or instruction is progressively weakened. The person with dementia may not recognize even their own relatives for who they are, less still the role, responsibility or authority of a professional seeking to help them. Indeed, their perception may be that well-intended approaches are uninvited, unnecessary and possibly dangerous.

Making sense of the environment poses similar difficulties. Even home may feel wrong and unfamiliar when your mind-set is that 'home' is where you lived 50 years ago with friends and family ungreyed by the time that has passed. And what are you to make of another place where people expect you to join in activities which are not your usual occupation and are not rewarded by a pay packet, or expect you to allow them involvement with the most personal of acts and then to get into bed at night and sleep without disturbance.

In extremes, people with dementia cannot comprehend words and cannot find the words they need to communicate their thoughts and wishes (receptive and expressive dysphasia). They may not understand what new activity they are being encouraged to perform, not recognizing objects, sounds, colours, even components of their own body (agnosia) or may be unable to initiate action despite their wish to co-operate (apraxia). Such impairment may be associated with misinterpretations of reality, misidentification of individuals or the suspicion that they have been replaced by doubles.

Characters on TV may be received and responded to as if whole and real and in the room, to be feared, respected or challenged. The individual may not recognize themselves in the mirror and deal with the image as a person, perhaps to be attacked, perhaps to be felt for, offered food and clothing.

The concentration span is impaired, as is the ability to persist with a task and to learn and rehearse new sequences of activity. Thinking reverts to the concrete, with flexibility and generalization of principle from the particular to similar challenges becoming difficult or impossible. This rigidity and narrowing of perspective may be associated with perseveration (repetition) on themes or individual acts. Pressure to expand the repertoire or increase flexibility may precipitate a catastrophic reaction of emotional distress or violence in reflex protest. It is simply too much and cannot be accommodated.

Non-cognitive symptoms (Allen et al. 1996; Burns, Jacoby and Levy 1990; Cummings et al. 1994; Hope et al. 1999)

Initiative, self-motivation and drive are diminished as a primary feature of dementia, particularly when the frontal lobe is affected by pathology. Monitoring of self-care, progress with the tasks necessary to maintain safety, cleanliness and dignity, is lost, leaving the individual at risk but apparently 'oblivious' and content to sit, lie or wander without sustained purpose.

In addition drive may be diminished as a secondary reaction to repeated failure and frustration when attempting to do what was previously possible. Thus the individual may stop trying, to avoid the pain of experiencing further failure or in acceptance that someone else will do what is necessary, more quickly and surely than they might.

Insight may be retained in some instances, usually when the syndrome is 'patchy' leaving some islands of fully functional brain cortex, as in vascular dementia. For the most part, however, in Alzheimer's disease and fronto-temporal dementia, insight is lost. It is necessary for others to identify problems and to make provision to compensate for deficiencies and hazards.

Burn holes in my pans? Not me.

Leave my front door wide open when I go shopping? Never.

Fall over when I stand? I don't think so. I'm better off without that **** walking frame to trip over.

Mood and mood control are often altered in dementia, anxiety and depression in some combination being the predominant features. These may be based in the neuro-chemical changes associated with neural loss in the degenerative process. They may represent return to a disorder evident earlier in life and possibly independent of the dementia. But they may arise in response to the difficulties dementia brings: loss of ability, loss of self-determination, loss of freedom and increasing dependency upon others.

Symptoms may include loss of confidence, loss of pleasure, self-deprecation, irritability, apathy, morbid preoccupations, thoughts of suicide or a wish for death, reduced interest in food, loss of weight, altered sleep.

Psychotic symptoms are less common but may occur. Illusions and hallucinations are usually visual, but may be auditory or involve bodily sensations of touch, heat, sexual interference etc. Visual hallucinations occur early and repeatedly in Lewy body dementia. They often feature children or colourful 'little people', sometimes attired in classical costumes. They may climb trees or float in silence through walls and furniture. In any other situation visual hallucinations should raise the suspicion of inter-current illness and delirium or an adverse effect of medication.

Delusional ideas may be based on hallucinatory experiences or arise as an apparently understandable response to failing cognition and altered circumstance:

I cannot find my purse. The family photograph has been moved from its usual place on the side-board. Ah! The neighbour, who pretends to be so caring and interested in my welfare, has stolen my key and has crept into my house to check and steal my most precious belongings.

I was quite happy and coping in my little house. I have been locked away in this Home. My daughter never comes to see me. She has taken possession of my house and is living there with her fancy man.

Appetite may be altered. Most usual is a waning of interest along with similar decline in enthusiasm for other activity. Less often appetite or desire for fluids is increased and may be insatiable. This latter can be hazardous raising the possibilities of choking, obesity or electrolyte imbalance. Preferences revert to simple tastes, especially for sweet things rather than a wholesome diet. In more deteriorated states individuals may find pleasure in odd or hazardous substances. One man produced an epidemic of swollen lips amongst his friends (other residents of a long-stay ward) by passing round tablets of soap to be sucked with apparent approval.

Sleep rhythm may change. Repeated short naps and a limited snooze at night time may suffice, but is not easy to accommodate in the routine of a family, nor even a care home which wants residents to sleep through the night shift. Episodic hypersomnia may occur, with three or more days of sleep alternating with similar periods of endless wakefulness. It is presumed that hypothalamic structures have been altered in such individuals. Narcolepsy may occur, but persistent energetic wakefulness is reported more often and causes great concern.

Altered motor activity is evident in many people with dementia and becomes more obvious as the condition progresses. Most people do less and sink deeper into their chairs with the associated hazards to muscle strength, joint function, venous circulation, balance, appetite, bowel function, mental liveliness and good humour and, eventually, skin quality and integrity.

The internal drive has gone. An external pacemaker is required. Others appear to do more, or at least don't stop walking about. Some have been life-long ramblers, shoppers and generally busy, busy bodies. They maintain their energy, may appear to require little nutriment and may demonstrate a degree of disinhibition in their restless determination to keep on the move. Combined with impaired concentration and distractability, the syndrome means it may be difficult to achieve constructive activity.

Disinhibition is indeed, perhaps the most notable and difficult of the non-cognitive symptoms of dementia. Loss of control of emotions may lead to tears and sobbing in response to minimal sadness. It may, alternatively, see the release of rage and verbal or physical aggression in response to minimal frustration or simply to fend off well-meaning and necessary attention to ensure cleanliness, dignity or safety. Sexual disinhibition may produce masturbation in public or in care situations and can lead to serious assaults on others if the boundaries of affectionate interaction between carer and cared for are breached. Simple loss of self-control may lead to embarrassment at the supermarket check-out when unnecessary items appear in the basket, or conversations with the store detective as shiny or sweet desirables are found concealed in a coat pocket or carried naively in the hand.

Factors and mechanisms leading to disability

There is much in the nature and symptomatology of dementia which predicts the emergence of disability. Yet some people remain lively and retain skills and joy despite the disorder, whilst others deteriorate apace. This may, in some instances, be because of the intrinsic attributes of the particular dementia. In addition it is appropriate to consider the disorder in context.

The individual in whom the dementia is occurring is 'host' to the process. It is a challenging and difficult role (Jolley and Jolley 1991; Kitwood 1997). There may be clues from previous struggles which will hint on the likely response and resolution to be achieved. Many have gone through difficult times earlier in life and emerged strong despite or because of the difficulties. Others may have had or engineered a more tranquil life style or found themselves overcome by previous stresses. Some may have experienced frank breakdowns. There may be clues in the family history to how such troubles will be met.

Around the individual is the assembly of immediate and wider family and friends and professional advisors and carers. These will, themselves, be in part product of the individual's personal style, interests and sensitivities as will be the domestic accommodation and other settings available to them. It is clear that dementia gives rise to the need for help, for prostheses to compensate for the losses of ability the neurological damage produces. It is from this circle of family, friends, professional carers and environments that prostheses must emerge and be fashioned.

- Will they be willing? (Let's hope so.)
- Will they be sufficiently resourced? (Family, friends and informal carers may have many other calls on their time. Professionals may be over-stretched.)
- Will they be well informed?
- Will they be supported throughout the long and changing demands of the process?

These prostheses will need to be strong and enduring. They will have to be re-jigged as conditions change, as the strength of other components of the support/therapeutic system wanes or falters. The best prostheses remain active. That is, they provide sufficient help to maintain safety and dignity, but offer time and encouragement, training and retraining so that the individual with dementia continues to do as much for self-care as is possible and as much for pleasure, entertainment and self-fulfilment as is possible. This way appetites, skills and joy are retained. The hazard, always, is to provide a sound but passive prosthesis, ensuring against obvious risks to safety, cleanliness and dignity, but not giving time to encourage the return of lost skills nor to prevent the atrophy of others.

Solutions in this mode may be quicker and appear cheaper in the short term. The cost in terms of lost opportunities for the individual with dementia is huge as they are ushered toward a time simply waiting for death. For the care agencies it is understood that the loss of one point on the Barthel scale of independence increases costs of caring by ten times that associated with a one point decline in cognitive function per se (Wolstenholme *et al.* 2002). Thus individuals with dementia may incur secondary losses of ability (losses not inevitable as consequence of neurological degeneration):

1. In their own homes because of lack of response to their needs. This may stem from failure to realize that there is anything wrong beyond the 'expected' decline of later life. It may be complicated by their rejection of help offered. It may be that neither family nor local services have sufficient or appropriate resource to help optimally.

2. In their own homes because the help given represents a passive prosthesis, fostering dependency.

3. At times of illness or in response to another crisis which leads to admission to hospital or other form of institutional care. People with dementia do not cope well with change. They may take longer than others to get over an illness. They certainly find it difficult to understand and adjust to relocation. Some give up the ghost and acquire disability and dependency from which they will not emerge without help. Others respond with anger in their bewilderment and find their vitality suppressed by medication as it cannot be coped with. Their dependency is thus further determined and complicated by the label of 'violent'.

Any of these scenarios can lead to a spiral of secondary and tertiary dependency. This can be reversed with vision and determination.

Long-term and family perspectives

Life with dementia may be brief but may continue for ten years or more. Life expectation amongst those known to have dementia has increased over recent decades. This is a positive commentary on improvements in understanding and care provided within every modality. It reflects that life with dementia may at times be tough, but it is worth the living (Jolley and Baxter 1997).

The strongest message to receive is that dementia takes away the strength, vision and certainty of the individual's personal control system. Someone else has to be at hand to trim the tiller if the journey is to proceed. 'Seeing people through' is one of the responsibilities Tom Arie identified for the early Psychogeriatric Services (Arie 1970). It should still be in all our mission statements. Yet specialist professional services function best when they become part of the family, complementing, advising and always respecting the plans, hopes and objectives of the individual within the context of their personal world.

Great difficulties can occur when individuals encounter services which deal with 'episodes' or 'cases', and whose performance is monitored and driven by turnover with little sensitivity to the long-term implications for the user and their family. Families and the best of primary care services (see Chapter 11) carry the knowledge which is necessary to interpret behaviour and disability in the life history and reasonable expectations of the individual. Their advocacy is essential so that objectives are set and realized which are based in the best interests of that individual, however humble and mundane those objectives might be. This is a process in which everyone has a role and within which the views and expertise of specialists, therapists, carers and people with dementia are to be used and weighed with equal respect and free from fear of criticism or disregard.

Life with dementia is worth living. Despite their dementia, individuals will have much to give. To do this they require help to maintain their best health, safety and dignity. They may need help to retain or regain mobility, continence and degrees of self-care. Then they can utilize their preserved skills and characteristics of wit and stories, affection and retort, song and smile to demonstrate and feel for themselves and for us that they are themselves and part of our family.

Summary

Older people are vulnerable to losing abilities beyond what is inevitable as a direct consequence of illness. This vulnerability is more marked in people with dementia. The symptoms of dementia include change and impairment in all aspects of mental function, they are not confined to problems of memory. Loss of vitality and self-determination are integral to dementia; primary or secondary depression is common. Behavioural reactions may frustrate attempts to help or be misinterpreted as malicious or informed rejection of appropriate therapy. Medication prescribed to suppress agitation or violence can confound recovery.

Lost abilities require compensation by prostheses. These should be flexible and responsive to changing needs and active in encouraging involvement of the individual with dementia as a contributor rather than passive recipient in the process. Individuals, family and professionals need to maintain a long-term perspective and commitment, setting goals which are reasonable and relevant to that individual and their position in their personal life-cycle and family.

References

Allen, N.H., Gordon, S., Hope, T. and Burns, A. (1996) 'The Manchester and Oxford Universities Scale for the Psychopathological Assessment of Dementia (MOUSEPAD).' *British Journal of Psychiatry 169*, 3, 293–307.

Arie, T. (1970) 'The first year of the Goodmayes psychiatric service for old people.' *Lancet ii*, 1179–1182.

Arie, T. and Jolley, D. (1998) 'Psychogeriatric services.' In R.C. Tallis, H.M. Fillitt and J.C. Brocklehurst (eds) *Brocklehurst's Textbook of Geriatric Medicine and Gerontology*. Edinburgh: Churchill-Livingstone, chapter 113, 1567–1573.

Black, D. and Jolley, D. (1990) 'Slow euthanasia? The deaths of psychogeriatric patients.' *British Medical Journal 300*, 1321–1323.

Burns, A., Jacoby, R. and Levy, R. (1990) 'Psychiatric phenomena in Alzheimer's disease I, II, III and IV.' *British Journal of Psychiatry 157*, 72–94.

Cummings, J.L., Mega, M., Gray, K., Rosenberg-Thompson, S., Carusi, D.A. and Gornbein, J. (1994) 'The Neuro-Psychiatric Inventory: A comprehensive assessment of psychopathology in dementia.' *Neurology 44*, 12, 2308–2314.

Hope, T., Keene, J., Fairburn, C., Jacoby, R. and McShane, R. (1999) 'Natural history of behavioural changes and psychiatric symptoms in Alzheimer's disease.' *British Journal of Psychiatry 174*, 6, 561–562.

Jolley, D. and Arie, T. (1978) 'Organisation of psychogeriatric services.' *British Journal of Psychiatry 132*, 1–11.

Jolley, D. and Baxter, D. (1997) 'Mortality in elderly patients with organic brain disorder.' *International Journal of Geriatric Psychiatry 12*, 12, 1174–1178.

Jolley, D. and Jolley, S. (1991) 'Psychiatry in the elderly.' In J. Pathy (ed) *Principles and Practice of Geriatric Medicine* (2nd edn). Chichester: John Wiley and Sons, 895–932.

Jorm, J.F., Korten, A. and Henderson, A.S. (1987) 'The prevalence of dementia: A quantitative integration of the literature.' *Acta Psychiatrica Scandinavica 76*, 465–478.

Kitwood, T. (1997) *Dementia Reconsidered: The Person Comes First*. Buckingham: Open University Press.

Lindesay, J., Marudkar, M., van Diepen, E. and Wilcocks, G. (2002) 'Memory Clinics.' *International Journal of Geriatric Psychiatry 17*, 1, 41–47.

Lishman, A.W. (1978) *Organic Psychiatry. The Psychological Consequences of Cerebral Disorder*. Oxford: Blackwell Scientific Publications.

Roth, M. (1955) 'The natural history of mental disorder in old age.' *Journal of Mental Science 101*, 281–301.

Townsend, P. (1962) *The Last Refuge*. London: Routledge, Kegan and Paul.

Warren, M. (1960) 'The evolution of Geriatric Medicine.' *Gerontologia Clinica 2*, 1–17.

Whitehead, T. (1978) *In the Service of Old Age* (2nd edn). Aylesbury: HM & M Publishers.

Wolstenholme, J., Fenn, P., Gray, A., Keene, J., Jacoby, R. and Hope, T. (2002) 'Estimating the relationship between disease progression and cost of care in dementia.' *British Journal of Psychiatry 181*, 36–42.

CHAPTER 3

The Historical Context of Rehabilitation and its Application to Dementia Care

Suzanne Cahill and Avril Dooley

Ask the average lay person on the street to provide a brief commentary about Alzheimer's disease in the context of rehabilitation and they will probably look at you as if you have ten heads. For certainly, until recently, the two concepts appeared incompatible, indeed mutually exclusive. On the one hand, Alzheimer's disease seemed to be synonymous with a notion of helplessness, hopelessness and therapeutic nihilism, 'the living death', whilst on the other, rehabilitation conjured up images of cure, recovery, empowerment and a return to full functioning capacity. Yet the term rehabilitation comes from the Latin words 're' and 'habilitare' meaning to 'again fit' or 'suit'. The Shorter Oxford Dictionary on Historical Principles defines the verb 'rehabilitate' as 'restore by formal act or declaration (a person degraded or attainted) to former privileges, rank and possession, to re-establish a person's good name or memory by authoritative pronouncement'. Indeed, as far back as 1847, to rehabilitate meant 'to re-establish the character or reputation of a person or thing' (Oxford University Press 1968). Drawing on these definitions, rehabilitation certainly does make sense in the context of dementia.

Why then has our understanding of this concept changed so significantly over time? Why and by whom have definitions of rehabilitation been hijacked? How can rehabilitation principles be usefully applied to improve services for older people with a dementia, indeed people who like all of us will ultimately face the reality of death? To address some of these questions and to understand the contemporary organization and purpose of rehabilitation it is useful first to trace the historical and ideological influences that shaped its development. The purpose of this chapter therefore is to define what is meant by the term rehabilitation and to detail more clearly how the concept has evolved over the years. It is suggested that whilst attempts to rehabilitate date back to Roman times, the two world wars were particularly instrumental in laying the foundation for a more worldwide rehabilitation movement. Various socio-political events including wars, medical and pharmacological advances, technology and social movements are identified as forces shaping the contemporary meaning and definition of rehabilitation.

A historical overview

Whilst most of us date the origin of rehabilitation back to the two world wars, curiously its history is considerably longer and extends over many centuries. Indeed, as far back as thousands of years ago, an Egyptian physician first documented his observations of a patient with a spinal cord injury when he detailed very thoroughly the patient's associated disability, a paralysis and urinary incontinence (Easton 1999). The earliest record of crutches on an Egyptian tomb is dated 2380 BC (Mumma 1987). Even as early as 400–300 BC, Hippocrates said 'exercise strengthens and inactivity wastes' (a pithy statement which continues to resonate for most of us today) when he documented the use of artificial limbs in patients with amputations (Mumma 1987).

Historically, the nursing profession has played a significant role in the promotion of rehabilitation concepts (Easton 1999). In the UK, for example, it was Florence Nightingale who in 1854 pioneered a significant role in the promotion of rehabilitation when she organized professional nursing training. According to some, she saved more lives through her novel rehabilitative techniques (using hygiene and basic rehabilitation principles practiced by the ancient Romans) than the entire British Medical Department at the time (Easton 1999). In the US, Isabel Hampton (1860–1910), another nurse educator, was also a leading pioneer of rehabilitation principles when she highlighted to her pupils the salience of cleanliness and asepsis to prevent secondary infections.

Whilst early records of such rehabilitation principles exist, it was not until during the two world wars that the most significant gains in rehabilitation were made by way of medical advancement and government legislation (Easton 1999). In the US, the First World War (1914–1918) resulted in a preponderance of war-time casualties, which generated a need to create services aimed at assisting disabled men to return to pre-war time functioning. Initially, services were of a custodial nature, confined exclusively to the armed forces and service delivery focused solely on physical rehabilitation or re-conditioning (Tomlinson 1943).

However, over time, the shortage of an active labour force combined with an increasing number of disabled servicemen returning from battlefields created the need to re-focus therapeutic interventions. Rehabilitation aims needed to be re-defined to include addressing the vocational needs of those wounded military personnel. In this regard, the setting up in 1917 of the American Red Cross Institute for Crippled and Disabled Men was instrumental and interestingly, the term rehabilitation replaced that of physical reconstruction of the disabled.

During the First World War, physicians who used therapy methods (called physical therapy physicians) and physical therapy technicians worked closely alongside each other. Physicians had lobbied and been successful in controlling both the medical and functional restoration of wartime victims and were considered the experts in charge of this area. In due course however, the Vocational Rehabilitation Act of 1920 transferred the responsibility of vocational rehabilitation away from the Surgeon General to non-physician-led federal departments, thereby diffusing physicians' power. Following this new piece of legislation, doctors struggling within their own profession joined forces with physical therapists to form the American College of Physical Therapy in 1921. Later, in 1929, the alliance between the two groups dissolved with the setting up of the American Physical Therapy Association. At this point in time it is said that physical therapists established interdependent relationships with physicians. Initially occupational therapists moved into psychiatric settings and tuberculosis sanitariums, but by 1923 they began to apply their skills in sensory and cognitive areas as complements to physical therapy and rehabilitation (Hoeman 2002). This marked the first move towards rehabilitating those who were not just bearers of physical impairments.

The Second World War brought further attention to the socio-political context of rehabilitation and its economic potential. The advent of sulfa drugs and other relevant medical advances meant that increasing numbers of wounded soldiers were returning from the battlefields to pose significant challenges to governments and society (Easton 1999). A key early champion of the principles of rehabilitation during this time was the American physician Harold Rusk, who through his pioneering work transformed public concern about the plight of the disabled into a more political campaign, lobbying for the rights of all those disadvantaged (not just wartime casualties) and for a rehabilitation movement (Rusk 1978). In 1943, the Vocational Rehabilitation Act was passed in the US which provided funding for training and research with the disabled. In 1947 Rusk brought the first Medical Rehabilitation services to an American hospital and some few years later (1958) was responsible for publishing 'Rehabilitation Medicine'. His strident championing is said to have touched the entire US nation, forcing people to recognize the limitations of attempting to heal the body alone (Easton 1999). His effort resulted in rehabilitation services being made available to civilians as well as military alike. Interestingly, Rusk, who in many ways was ahead of his time, challenged the dominant ideology of the period by subscribing to a social model of health and illness which saw the importance of looking beyond the signs and symptoms of an illness towards understanding the uniqueness of the individual and the salience of his or her quality of life.

In the US, the year 1938 saw the setting up of the American Academy of Physical Medicine and Rehabilitation and this was soon followed by the establishment of the American Board of Physical Medicine and Rehabilitation in 1947. However, it was not until the mid 1950s that rehabilitation became fully accepted as a viable medical speciality in its own right and the medical view of disability has up until recently held dominance in most professional discourse and has remained highly influential in shaping the development of rehabilitation services. Accordingly the medical profession has long been regarded as expert in diagnosis and assessment. The rehabilitation professionals – parapetic staff, including physiotherapists, occupational therapists and speech and language therapists – have been promoted as experts to treat and to respond to complex problems of impairment.

Within this socio-political context, and broadly speaking, rehabilitation has moved from the 1950s where the focus was predominantly on surgical restoration for road traffic accidents and orthopaedic patients (Piercy 1956), to stroke rehabilitation in the 1960s (Licht 1973), to cardiac rehabilitation in the 1970s (Carson *et al.* 1973) and, although almost non-existent in the early 1970s, rehabilitation in the area of brain injury has progressed significantly over the past 20 years (Giles 1994). More recently cognitive rehabilitation has become an emerging speciality with the medical and neuro-psychological fields (Clare and Woods 2001). Historically, therefore, rehabilitation has tended to be owned by medicine and has emerged largely as a result of scientific and medical advancement. It was traditionally seen as a way to restore disabled people and maintain productivity in response to problems associated with impairments. More recently, however, demographic and other socio-political changes have resulted in the concept of rehabilitation being re-cast. The following section will discuss some of the possible reasons why such changes may have come about.

An emerging new understanding of the meaning of rehabilitation

A series of factors has brought about the need to re-conceptualize the term rehabilitation and re-cast its meaning. One such factor has been population ageing – now a widespread phenomenon in the Western world. Fifty years ago, when average life expectancy was significantly lower than it is today, conventional models of rehabilitation underpinned by Positivism and looking at outcome measures such as functional ability, return to work, survival or illness recurrence made a lot more sense than they do now. Longevity paralleled with an increase in medical and technological advances in health and social care has meant traditional models of rehabilitation are now inadequate to meet older people's multiple diverse needs. Accordingly, rehabilitation programmes have had to adjust to accommodate. Population ageing, for example, has meant an increase in the prevalence of chronic health conditions which are sometimes lifelong and require the setting up of both short term and long term rehabilitative goals (Nolan 2001). The shift from acute to more long term chronic health problems has in no small way challenged the traditional model of rehabilitation.

Another significant development impacting on changes in definitions of rehabilitation can be seen in the huge contribution recently made to this body of literature (Chamberlain 1992; Fitzpatrick 1996; McLellan 1991; Nocon and Baldwin 1998; Renwick and Friefild 1996). Recent writers now argue that the topic of rehabilitation has over the years been fraught with methodological problems due to a lack of standardization in definition and that the commonest incorrect assumption is that rehabilitation is time-limited and has a clear end point (Young 1996). Those who critique current rehabilitation practices argue that not infrequently the views of 'patients' are neglected (Ebrahim 1994) and that therapeutic goals tend to be driven by economists and result in quantifiable outcomes which have a measurement orientation and may be of little relevance to the actual people concerned, those with a disability (Nolan 2001). A 'creaming off' process of rehabilitation is also said to exist wherein the emphasis has been placed on selecting clients who give greater promise for desired changes (Coudroglou 1984). Those who advocate the need to re-conceptualize rehabilitation exhort us to look beyond measures such as survival and illness recurrence and move towards a model of rehabilitation which focuses on whether a person's life accords with his or her wishes (Ebrahim 1994) and a system which sustains a positive sense of direction in the face of major losses (Nolan 2001).

The increase in the incidence and prevalence of dementia across the world coupled with the pioneering and revolutionary work of the late Tom Kitwood who critiqued in depth the bio-medical model approach towards understanding dementia and re-conceptualized it to be regarded as a disability (Kitwood 1997) has also provided a firm theoretical basis for the application of rehabilitation principles. Kitwood's major thesis is that a person with dementia is not just disadvantaged cognitively and physically due to the neurological impairment but may also be excessively disabled due to adverse psychological social and environmental influences (Kitwood 1997). The environment, he maintained, often constituted a malignant social psychology which serves to dehumanize the individual, thereby accentuating the level of disability. He argued that people with dementia remain primarily social beings who continue to live in social worlds.

Their past experiences, roles and relationships greatly determine their behaviour. He posits that while the neurological impairment experienced in dementia may not be easily treated, other non-medical factors may respond well to psycho-social interventions. Accordingly, the individual's experience of dementia may be largely contingent on the quality of care received. In his careful social deconstruction of dementia, Kitwood demonstrates the potential for rehabilitation in dementia care and the possibility of a better quality of life for those affected by this disability. Kitwood's theoretical analysis of dementia has been revolutionary in laying the framework for the merger of these two important areas of practice and thinking, rehabilitation and dementia.

The recent worldwide increases in the detection and diagnosis of vascular and mixed dementia largely aided by rapid and significant advances in modern medicine and technology including the advent of MRI and SPECT scanning has shed increasing light on the potential people with dementia have for rehabilitation. There is some evidence available from the systolic hypertension in Europe (Syst-Eur) study which shows that cardiovascular risk factors such as hypertension are associated with vascular and mixed dementia (Forette et al. 2002). Results from multi-centred trials show that even in patients who have had strokes or TIAS, secondary prevention as reflected in the subsequent control of these cardiovascular risk factors reduces the risk of further events quite significantly and consequently slows down the pathways leading to more severe dementia (Sandercock 2003; Tzourio and Anderson 2000).

Theoretically, indeed, it is said that vascular dementia may be one of the dementias most amenable to treatment and to risk factor intervention (Sandercock 2003). The rehabilitation of people with vascular and mixed dementia forces us to move beyond the notion of 'restoration of function' to include the resolution of non-biological or social issues. The cessation of smoking, moderate alcohol consumption, regular exercise, blood pressure monitoring and a balanced diet complete with reduced saturated fat and salt intake, are each important social areas lending themselves well to rehabilitation principles. The great advantage of thinking rehabilitation and disability in the context of dementia is that it forces us to think about people's rights to services and generates a sense of hope, creating a vision for the future.

New anti-dementia drugs

Finally, the advent of the new anti-dementia drugs developed over the last decade (including Donepezil, Rivastigmine and Galantamine) is yet another social force causing us to think rehabilitation in the context of dementia. Dementia attacks the cholinergic system in the brain – a system vital for memory and learning –

and these anti-dementia drugs have been designed to protect the latter through boosting levels of acetycholine, a brain chemical considered vital for nerve cells to communicate and known to become depleted in dementia, (Burns, Page and Winter 2001). It is important to remember that anti-dementia drugs do not cure dementia or impact on the basic disease destructive mechanism, but rather slow down the cognitive deterioration. The medication has been shown to have a 30 to 40 per cent success rate in certain sub-groups. For the person with dementia, the advent of these anti-dementia drugs may result in more honesty and frankness in doctor-patient relationships, since the person being prescribed the medication is more likely to be told why such an intervention is needed. The advent of such drugs offers the individual with dementia the prospect of rehabilitation and most importantly hope for the future.

Summary

This chapter has attempted to trace some of the historical and socio-political events (wars, medical advances, social movements and technology) which have helped to shape the contemporary meaning, organization and purpose of rehabilitation programmes. It has been shown how although early rehabilitation efforts date back to Roman times, the two world wars were instrumental in spawning rehabilitation principles and laying the foundation for how the concept is perceived today. The chapter has also detailed some of the changes emerging in our understanding of the term rehabilitation (Nolan 2001) and put forward reasons why these may have come about.

Currently there exists no unified model of rehabilitation, rather theories from a wide variety of disciplines contribute to a knowledge base, which provides a framework to inform and broaden the scope of rehabilitation practice. The shift from the more traditional view, where rehabilitation was seen as a finite time-limited individualistic process, to the more contemporary view where a temporal eclectic approach is taken (Nolan 2001) and where outcomes are measured not only in economic terms but by subjective and contextual indicators has been noted. The chapter also drew on key principles in rehabilitation and demonstrated how each can usefully be explicated and applied to best practice in dementia care.

Of particular note when researching material for this chapter was the fact that there appears to be a paucity of literature on the topic of rehabilitation and dementia. Indeed, from several database searches undertaken, most of the published works on the topic tend to focus on cognitive rehabilitation (Clare and Woods 2001). The absence of a specific literature linking together the two key concepts of rehabilitation and dementia is an exciting finding as it offers an opportunity for all of us dementia enthusiasts to be creative, to trailblaze and to draw on the more contemporary principles of rehabilitation to attempt to change practice and improve the quality of life of all those diagnosed with a cognitive impairment.

The literature notes that several rehabilitation processes have emerged not as a result of strategic planning but due to health professionals' own enthusiasm for particular practices (Beardshaw 1988). It is timely, therefore, that efforts now proceed to test out new emerging principles on rehabilitation in dementia care practice, thereby promoting more independent living for people with this disability. It is timely too that efforts are made to forge links between thinking and practice and to merge these two very important bodies of literature on dementia and on rehabilitation, thereby advancing the dementia movement yet another step forward.

References

Beardshaw, V. (1988) *Last on the List: Community Services for People with Physical Disabilities.* London: King's Fund Institute.

Burns, A., Page, S. and Winter, J. (2001) *Alzheimer's Disease and Memory Loss Explained.* Middlesex: Altman Publishing.

Carson, P., Neophytou, M., Tucker, H. and Simpson, T. (1973) 'Exercise programme after myocardial infarction.' *British Medical Journal 4*, 213–216.

Chamberlain, M.A. (1992) 'The metamorphosis of physical medicine?' *Journal of the Royal Society of Medicine 85*, 131–135.

Clare, L. and Woods, B. (2001) 'Editorial: A role for cognitive rehabilitation in dementia care.' In L. Clare and B. Woods (eds) *A Special Issue of the Journal of Cognitive Rehabilitation in Dementia 11*, 3, 193–196.

Coudroglou, A. (1984) 'Disability: the view from social policy.' *Rehabilitation Literature 45*, 358–361.

Easton, K. (1999) *Gerontological Rehabilitation Nursing.* Philadelphia: W.B. Saunders.

Ebrahim, S. (1994) 'The goals of rehabilitation for older people.' *Reviews in Clinical Gerontology 4*, 2, 93–96.

Fitzpatrick, R. (1996) 'Patient centred approaches to the evaluation of health care.' In K.W.M. Fulford, S. Ersser and T. Hope (eds) *Essential Practice in Patient Centred Care.* Oxford: Blackwell Science.

Forette, F., Seux, M.L., Staessen, J.A., Thijs, L., Babarskiene, M.R., Babeanu, S., Bossini, A., Fagard, R., Gil-Extremera, B., Laks, T., Kobalava, Z., Sarti, C., Tuomilehto, J., Vanhanen, H., Webster, J., Yodfat, Y. and Birkenhager, W.H. (2002) 'Systolic hypertension in Europe investigators. The prevention of dementia with antihypertensive treatment: New evidence from the systolic hypertension in Europe (Syst-Eur) study.' *Archives Internal Medicine 162*, 18, 2046–2052.

Giles, G.M. (1994) 'Why provide community support for persons with brain injury?' *American Journal of Occupational Therapy 48*, 295–296.

Hoeman, S. (2002) *Rehabilitation Nursing Process, Applications and Outcomes* (3rd edn). London: Mosby.

Licht, S. (1973) 'Stroke: A history of its rehabilitation: The Walter Zeiter Lecture.' *Archives of Physical Medicine Rehabilitation 54*, 1, 10–8 passim.

Kitwood, T. (1997) *Dementia Reconsidered: The Person Comes First.* Buckingham: Open University Press.

McLellan, D.L. (1991) 'Functional recovery and the principles of disability medicine.' In M. Swash and J. Oxbury (eds) *Clinical Neurology 1*, 768–790.

Mumma, C.M. (1987) *Rehabilitation Nursing: Concepts and Practice* (2nd edn). Evanston, IL: Rehabilitation Nursing Foundation.

Nocon, A. and Baldwin, S. (1998) *Towards a Rehabilitation Policy: A Review of the Literature.* London: Kings Fund.

Nolan, M. (2001) 'Acute and rehabilitative care for older people.' In M. Nolan, S. Davies and G. Grant (eds) *Working with Older People and their Families. Key Issues in Policy and Practice.* Buckingham: Open University Press.

Piercy, W. (1956) *Report of the Committee of Enquiry on the Rehabilitation, Training and Resettlement of Disabled Persons.* London: Parliamentary Papers (Cmd. 9883).

Renwick, R. and Friefild, S. (1996) 'Quality of life and rehabilitation.' In R. Renwick, I. Brown and M. Nagler (eds) *Quality of Life in Health Promotion: Conceptual Approaches, Issues and Applications.* Thousand Oaks, CA: Sage.

Rusk, H.A. (1978) 'The 1977 Walter Zeiter Lecture. Rehabilitation medicine: Knowledge in search of understanding.' *Archives of Physical Medicine Rehabilitation 59*, 156–160.

Sandercock, P.A.G. (2003) 'Should I start all my ischaemic stroke and TIA patients on a statin, an ACE inhibitor, a diuretic, and aspirin today?' *Journal of Neurological Neurosurgery Psychiatry 74*, 1461–1464.

Tomlinson, G. (1943) *Report on the Inter Departmental Committee on the Rehabiliation and Resettlement of Disabled Persons.* 6415. London: HSMO.

Tzourio, C. and Anderson, C. (2000) 'Blood pressure reduction and risk of dementia in patients with stroke: Rationale of the dementia assessment in PROGRESS (Perindopril Protection Against Recurrent Stroke Study) PROGRESS Management Committee.' *Journal of Hypertension Supplement 18*, 1, S21–24.

Young, J. (1996) 'Caring for older people: Rehabilitation and older people.' *British Medical Journal 313*, 7058, 677–681.

CHAPTER 4

Intermediate Care: The New Pathway to Rehabilitation or Widening the Chasm?

Kate Read

Other chapters in this book identify the benefits of a rehabilitative approach in caring for older people with dementia, but have also demonstrated that few people are able to access services with that focus. When intermediate care made its appearance on the English stage it presented a great opportunity to increase the drive towards rehabilitation in mental health care for older people. It is timely now to look at developments since the first funding became available. This chapter seeks to identify the potential of intermediate care to support people with dementia but also to explore some of the constraints which have made it a scarce resource for people with dementia. It will conclude by suggesting possible models of service.

What is intermediate care?

Intermediate care is viewed by many as a subset of rehabilitation, focused on short term transitional support, with the therapeutic aim of improving health and function to maximize independence. One of the Standards of the National Service Framework for Older People is dedicated to intermediate care and was explicit in its requirement that:

> Older People will have access to a new range of intermediate care services at home or in designated care settings, to promote their independence by providing enhanced services from the NHS and councils to prevent unnecessary hospital admission and effective rehabilitation services to enable early discharge

from hospital and to prevent premature or unnecessary admission to long term residential care. (Department of Health 2001a, p.41)

Thus the aims of intermediate care became clear – it was about improving hospital discharge through rehabilitation, reducing avoidable hospital admission and avoiding long term care.

Intermediate care was specifically defined as services which met all of the following criteria:

- focus on early discharge or avoidable admission to acute in-patient or long term residential care

- comprehensive assessment leading to active treatment and rehabilitation

- maximizing independence

- interventions no longer than six weeks, often one to two weeks

- multidisciplinary.

The aspiration of intermediate care was summarized as 'an opportunity to maximise people's physical functioning, build confidence, re-equip them with the skills they need to live safely and independently at home, and plan any on-going support needed' (Department of Health 2001a, p.45).

And in that one word 'physical' the difficulties which have surrounded rehabilitation for older people with dementia were compounded for the next two years.

What prompted intermediate care?

Demographic factors

Probably the key driver to intermediate care was a demographic one with its financial implications for the health services. People aged over 70 use 40 per cent of hospital beds and half of those older hospitalized people are likely to be readmitted within 18 months of discharge. (Steiner 1997). Thus the projection of a 50 per cent rise in the over 80s between 1995 and 2025 has potentially profound consequences for health and social care resources.

The case for preventative and rehabilitative services was most convincingly made by the Audit Commission in 1997 with its conceptualization of the 'vicious circle'. It identified that lack of investment in prevention and rehabilitation resulted in higher spending on inpatients, which in turn reduced the capacity to invest in prevention and rehabilitation, thus the cycle of escalating demand on inpatient services was perpetuated.

Policy

The Department of Health's National Bed Inquiry (2000a) found that 20 per cent of bed days for older people were probably inappropriate and unnecessary if alternative facilities were available. This was quickly followed by a circular from the Department of Health (2001b) giving guidance on intermediate care, upon which the National Service Framework (NSF) subsequently expanded. Critically the NHS Plan (Department of Health 2000b) signalled new investment in intermediate care, which it later became clear was the only significant funding for services to accompany the older people's National Service Framework. Sadly the initial guidance of intermediate care was widely interpreted as excluding older people with dementia. Thus the second set of guidance published by the Department of Health in 2002 was much welcomed for its explicit statement specifically including older people with mental illness or dementia.

Finance

The implications of not intervening in the 'vicious circle' were manifestly important. In recent years health and social care managers have been required to focus much of their energy on three key questions:

1. How to stop the escalating use of Accident and Emergency units, leading to 'trolley waits'?

2. How to stop 'bed blocking'?

3. How to stop inappropriate residential/nursing home admissions consuming social services budgets and creating another raft of dependent people?

Intermediate care was viewed as the potential answer to each of these questions and the ever demanding budgetary constraints. The new money which accompanied its introduction paved the way to a large number of developments.

Practice

Developments in practice were also significant catalysts. In particular advances in technology, nursing and medicine enabled more people with complex needs to be supported at home. Likewise patient choice and the aspiration of seamless care create a context into which intermediate care can make a significant contribution, and, lastly, early evaluations have given positive encouragement to further development.

The case for including people with dementia

The likelihood of developing dementia increases with age, with over 20 per cent of people over 80 having dementia (Audit Commission 2000). Thus it is estimated that by 2050 there will be 1.2 million people with dementia in the UK. If people with dementia are excluded from key strategies like intermediate care the strategy will fail to address its underpinning drivers.

Estimates suggest that 15 to 20 per cent of older inpatients have dementia in addition to their presenting difficulty. One factor, which bedevils both accurate estimates and effective care, is the lack of mental health expertise in acute general hospitals. The Change Agent Team autumn roadshow, supported by anecdotal evidence, suggests that difficulty in placing people with dementia is a significant factor in delayed discharge from hospital. And it is widely recognized that hospital admission is doubly traumatic for someone with dementia, who will struggle with the dementia-unfriendly surroundings as well as disorientation from dislocation from familiar people and environment which then compounds confusion and puts a return home in further doubt. These are the very people who go directly to a nursing home.

A report by the Nuffield Institute for Health (2002) found evidence that people with dementia were most likely to have a prolonged hospital stay and a delayed discharge due to placement difficulties. So addressing their needs is vital to tackling the problems and giving them a better experience.

Forget Me Not (Audit Commission 2000) estimated that 33 per cent of people in care homes have dementia and from the NSF (Department of Health 2001a) we know that 63 per cent of those entering nursing homes and 43 per cent entering residential care do so directly from hospital. If intermediate care fails to address the rehabilitative needs of people with dementia the primary targets of improving discharge and intervening to prevent inappropriate admission will not be met.

The NSF recognizes that rehabilitation can improve cognitive functioning, thus a rationale for exclusion based on lack of evidence of effectiveness is flawed. The later guidance on intermediate care is very specific in debunking such arguments: 'the evidence is that they can benefit equally well' (Department of Health 2002a, p.12).

Supporters of the inclusion of people with dementia have cited the evidence of a study by Huusko *et al.* in 2000. This demonstrated that people with a hip fracture and dementia can successfully be rehabilitated. Moreover, in the one year follow-up study significantly less people with dementia in the rehabilitation group had gone into institutional care – not only did they return home, they stayed there!

Fundamentally a positive approach to addressing mental health issues is a crucial factor in successful rehabilitation. And, less positively, it is recognized that caring for people with dementia who have a concomitant physical problem strains the resources of an acute ward, creates frustration for staff and is frequently a frightening experience for the person.

Opportunity or obstacle?

In the early development of intermediate care many services excluded people with dementia, citing that the six-week maximum intervention set out in the criteria was too short for effective therapeutic work with people with dementia. This has some validity. But less valid but also frequently stated was the view that cognitive impairment necessarily led to inability to follow a therapeutic regime and implied poor motivation. Early writing on intermediate care reinforced this perspective: 'for many intermediate care options, the people best able to benefit are cognitively intact, non-institutionalised and... They have to be motivated' (Steiner 1997, p.54). Likewise commentaries have omitted or could not find services which addressed dementia.

The tendency of early services to gravitate to physical rehabilitation and implicitly if not explicitly exclude people with dementia is regrettable, but within the pressured health and care context at the time it is partly understandable. It is challenging to achieve the rehabilitation of someone with dementia in six weeks. But in a climate of targets requiring demonstrable success, the temptation was also to work with people needing physical rehabilitation, who were more likely to show evidence of quick gains and predictable outcomes and even demonstrable financial savings.

The other key factor that led to people with dementia being excluded appears to be lack of mental health expertise in all parts of the system. People were sent to hospital because primary care staff did not feel competent to address the complicating factor of dementia. Once in hospital many acute staff lacked the training to recognize or work with the dementia and those who assessed for discharge tended towards the least risky option of institutional care. The final confounding factor was that the intermediate care services themselves were set up with staff and environments focusing on physical needs, so lacked confidence to work with dementia and were often unable to access specialist staff in mental health services for older people. Mental health expertise was rarely specified in the initial commissioning process so the teams themselves could scarcely be blamed for not addressing dementia.

What makes intermediate care work

The second and detailed set of guidance on intermediate care that came out in 2002 (Department of Health) very helpfully set out the guiding principles as:

- person centred care
- whole system working
- timely access to specialist care
- promoting health and active life. (p.7)

These principles apply equally to care for people with dementia. So an intermediate care service which genuinely follows these principles is well set to meet the needs of people with dementia as well as older people with other challenges.

However the essential first step is to ensure that the assessment which initiates the intermediate care service is timely and effective in recognizing and addressing the needs of a person with dementia. Sadly, to date, that key has frequently been missing and people with dementia have failed to get through the door. Many hopes are pinned on the single assessment process, but early pilots suggest that further work will be required to bring mental health into a pivotal role.

Potentially intermediate care's greatest contribution lies in its function as a bridge between existing complex and fragmented services. For an older person in crisis the responses are often compartmentalized, leading to a series of interventions by different teams and often several moves (see Figure 4.1).

Whilst there have been creative efforts to set up services which bridge the gap between primary and secondary care the outcome has often felt, from the older person's experience, less of a supportive mechanism, more of an obstacle course. It takes little imagination to see how this would be experienced by a person with dementia. Carers have given compelling accounts of the disorientation and distress which rapidly changing locations and personnel have wrought. If the service is to work effectively for people with dementia it cannot be another pier for that bridge but rather the mortar which creates the linkage between the existing blocks, or better still, bonds services together in a permanent way which reduces the complexity for the person but also makes the structure more robust – the more seams the greater potential for a weakness to develop!

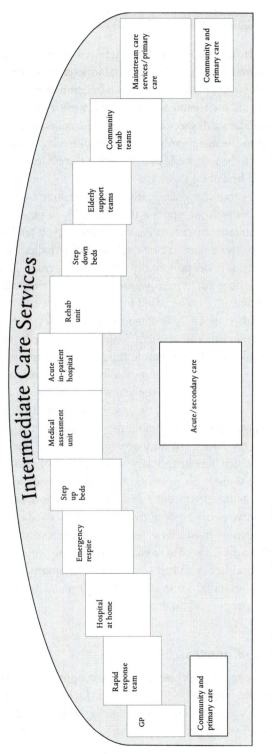

Intermediate Care Services

| Rapid response team | Step up beds | Medical assessment unit | Acute in-patient hospital | Rehab unit | Step down beds | Elderly support teams | Community rehab teams | Mainstream care services/primary care |

GP

Emergency respite

Hospital at home

Community and primary care

Acute/secondary care

Community and primary care

Figure 4.1 Spectrum of care supported by Intermediate Care

A thousand flowers

The Department of Health's 2002 guidance referred to intermediate care as 'A thousand flowers have bloomed'. There are good examples of services which divert people with dementia from unnecessary admission or enable return home, as the Nuffield Institute for Health found in their workshops (2002). To date, however, they tend to be small specimen blooms with roots in specialist services rather than integral to the main gardens. Another difficulty at this point is that many services are yet to be fully evaluated, therefore the evidence base is limited. There is still much to be done.

The key challenge to intermediate care services wishing to provide dementia-appropriate services is to incorporate the principles of good dementia care into the value base of intermediate care. Person-centred care is readily assimilated but other facets of positive dementia care could be more challenging. For example, people with dementia suffer profoundly if moved unnecessarily, continuity of care is important. This does not fit readily into criteria for intermediate care units, although the development of home based intermediate care services could promote positive dementia care. There is much to be gained from bringing mental health skills into intermediate care services. Similarly there are benefits in bringing intensive interventions, which promote the greatest independence possible, into mainstream dementia care. All could gain from this approach.

Probably the greatest challenge to the majority of intermediate care services is also the greatest challenge in dementia care. How are we to engage primary care? To date there have been few champions for prioritizing in primary care, and similarly GPs have in the main been wary of intermediate care, feeling that it left them with problems which have historically been the remit of secondary services. To gain primary care support for dementia-focused intermediate care will be a serious challenge. But the intermediate care/primary care interface is hugely valuable and whilst services have tended to focus on the secondary care interface there is much to be gained from renewed energy in relationship building with primary care. Mechanisms are needed to ensure that appropriate services are commissioned to meet local needs and this will need champions in Primary Care Trusts who will own the mental health issues and understand the potential impact on the lives of older people and their carers.

Evolving models of practice

To date three strategic approaches have evolved to support people with dementia needing intermediate care. The first has its location and management arrangements firmly within specialist services for older people with mental illness. They are usually small projects specifically for people with dementia and have a tightly defined role. Such projects include specific intermediate care units for people with dementia or the creation of a team with a specific remit to provide a comprehensive assessment with initial therapy and care which avoids inappropriate admission. The second approach has been to recruit mental health professionals as core members of generic intermediate care services, thereby enabling the team to confidently accept people with dementia.

The third approach is to develop mental health expertise in all intermediate care practitioners and indeed the secondary and primary care referrers. The resources required to do this effectively are extensive and it is therefore a less developed approach, although the potential impact of such widely available expertise is great. There is some concern that the skills needed to work rehabilitatively with people with dementia are very specialized and it is unlikely that the level of investment required to 'skill up' generic services could be found, which could dissipate the effectiveness. It also requires robust liaison arrangements to access specialist support when required.

The other burning debate in intermediate care for people with dementia is the dilemma of community-based services or location in specialist units. Given the established principle that people with dementia can struggle if moved unnecessarily and that there is some evidence for the effectiveness of community-based solutions (Nuffield Institute for Health 2002), the weight seems to lean towards community-based options where possible. However, given the number of moves often experienced in acute hospitals and the strong evidence base of the direct slide towards nursing home care from hospital, a specialist unit which can successfully give people with dementia an understanding place to recover functioning and ultimately return home has its place. Small domestic-styled units adjacent to generic intermediate care may be a strategy. The challenge will be to bring the principles of good dementia care and supportive environments into generic intermediate care units which are likely to be places of transition and intensive therapy.

There appear to be a range of models developing, all with potential:

- Liaison teams to support nursing or residential home staff aimed at preventing people who present challenges from being moved unnecessarily into acute hospital care.

- Specialist teams supporting people with dementia intensively in their own home to prevent an avoidable admission or facilitate discharge.

- Specialist input into generic home based intermediate care services.

- Specialist dementia assessment teams who can comprehensively assess and make initial interventions at points of crises and set up ongoing maintenance care plans.

- Working with family carers to enhance support when their person with dementia develops a physical illness – the interplay between the physical difficulties and the dementia symptoms is often the 'last straw'.
- Working in acute settings to minimize disorientation and maintain independent functioning and contribute mental health expertise to the discharge assessment process.
- Specialist dementia intermediate care units.
- Generic intermediate care units with dementia specific expertise.

Where next?

People with dementia have needs which could benefit from intermediate care services, however, the approach to delivering that service will have to be sensitive to the dementia factors and therefore will be different. The cost of not including people with dementia is high both in terms of quality of life for the person and their family and also in financial terms for the whole health and social care system.

There are models of good practice and teams doing hugely effective work. But it seems that these are isolated pockets, frequently battling to establish the integration and flexibility needed. The key will lie in creating the will to work creatively in partnership with colleagues and systems in a way that is 'out of the box' of established practice.

The Change Agent Team (in a series of roadshows in autumn 2002) presented two challenges to local services and commissioners:

What services do you need to have in place so that:

- no one is admitted to hospital inappropriately
- no older person admitted to hospital from their own home is discharged directly to long term care in a nursing or residential home. (Department of Health 2002b)

The real challenge is to make that thinking and planning genuinely inclusive of people with dementia.

References

Audit Commission (1997) *Coming of Age.* London: Audit Commission.

Audit Commission (2000) *Forget Me Not.* London: Audit Commission.

Department of Health (2000a) *National Bed Inquiry (NBI). Shaping the Future NHS: Long Term Planning for Hospitals and Related Services.* London: Department of Health.

Department of Health (2000b) *The NHS Plan: A Plan for Investment, a Plan for Reform.* London: Department of Health.

Department of Health (2001a) *National Service Framework for Older People.* London: Department of Health.

Department of Health (2001b) *Intermediate Care.* Circular HSC 2001/01: LAC 2001.

Department of Health (2002a) *Intermediate Care: The Way Forward.* London: Department of Health.

Department of Health (2002b) *Change Agent Team Autumn 2002 Roadshow.* www.dh.gov.uk

Huusko, T., Karppi, P., Avikainen, V., Kaulianen, H. and Sulkava, R. (2000) 'Randomised clinically controlled trial of intensive geriatric rehabilitation in patients with hip fracture: subgroup analysis of patients with dementia.' *British Medical Journal 7269,* 321, 1107–1111.

Nuffield Institute for Health (2002) *Exclusivity or Exclusion.* Leeds: Nuffield.

Steiner, A. (1997) *Intermediate Care: A Conceptual Framework and Review of the Literature.* London: Kings Fund.

CHAPTER 5

Rehabilitation for People with Dementia: Pointers for Practice from the Evidence Base

Gail Mountain

Introduction

Rehabilitation is not a new concept. However, policy awareness of the potential of rehabilitation both in terms of improving the quality of life of vulnerable people and reducing expenditure on residential care is relatively recent (Department of Health (DH) 2000; DH 2001a). Even so, attention has tended to concentrate upon those with physical frailty and/or physical illness and consequent disabilities rather than those with mental health problems (DH 2001b). The rehabilitation needs of older people with mental health problems, including dementia, tend to have been overlooked (Nuffield Institute for Health 2002). It is only now that interest in this area of practice is being generated within the wider health and social care community.

This chapter critiques some of the evidence to support rehabilitation with people with dementia, and out of this some pointers for service development and practice are identified.

Understanding the key terms for the search

The starting point for searching for evidence was to explicate the interpretations that can be placed upon the key terms to determine the parameters of the search.

Rehabilitation

Rehabilitation is a complex construct with a range of understandings. It can be applied to care processes as well as services. This complexity was clearly illustrated during a seminar on rehabilitation with professionals held at the King's Fund in 1996:

> ...while it was clear that while everyone knew what he or she meant by rehabilitation, their interpretation was not necessarily shared by others. Meanings differ according to what is involved, who benefits, who provides opportunities for rehabilitation and where. (Robinson and Batstone 1996, p.4)

The recent, enhanced interest in rehabilitation has served to increase this complexity. Mountain (2001) noted that different interpretations are being adopted by health and social services; namely medical and social rehabilitation. Furthermore, recent policy initiatives have raised the rehabilitative profile of services that aim to promote social inclusion as well as those concerned with assisting people to attain maximum independence.

As Robinson and Batstone (1996) confirmed, different professional groups have established alternative interpretations of what rehabilitation is and the interventions that it includes. One way of achieving consensus is through the World Health Organization's International Classification of functioning, disability and health (ICF) (World Health Organization 2001). The ICF acknowledges the interaction between the individual and the personal and environmental contexts within which they live, seeking to integrate medical and social models. The terms 'body functions' and 'structures', 'activities' and 'participation' have replaced 'impairment', 'disability' and 'handicap'.

The literature specific to people with Alzheimer's disease uncovers further understandings of rehabilitation. The importance of activity in enhancing quality of life, as well as aspects like maintenance of dignity, relationships and psychological well-being, is promoted (Perrin 1997). The concept of personhood has also been described in relation to people with dementia. This was promoted through the work of the Bradford Dementia group (Benson 2000; Kitwood 1997). Personhood enables a positive view of people with dementia, with a focus upon the whole person, drawing upon their strengths as well as taking into account declining abilities in some areas. There is a need for enhanced verbal and non verbal communication (Allan 2001; Kitwood 1993).

The gulf that can exist between the beliefs of workers dedicated to the rehabilitation and care of people with dementia and those working in other forms of rehabilitation service is exemplified by the following quote from an occupational therapist working in a home treatment team for people with dementia:

Unfortunately, people with dementia are sometimes seen as 'unsuitable for rehab' … This can arise if dementia is seen one-sidedly as a process of degeneration, or if rehabilitation is seen largely in terms of functional performance or simplistic notions of independence rather than of facilitating renewed personhood or well-being. (Wey 2002, p.30)

This brief overview confirms that an exploratory approach has to be adopted to determine the range of interventions and services that might be deemed to be rehabilitative in the context of the needs of people with dementia.

People with dementia

The expression 'people with dementia' includes younger people with early onset Alzheimer's disease as well as those who are very old, therefore representing a highly heterogeneous group. The circumstances that people with dementia find themselves in also embraces a multitude of possibilities, like degree of physical and mental impairment, living circumstances and available networks of care. Rehabilitation services and interventions have to take account of this individuality. This review was not limited to specific groups of people with dementia, but it did exclude those with a predominant physical illness (such as stroke) and a secondary diagnosis of dementia.

Carers of people with dementia

The carers of people with dementia are pivotal in that they can help to maintain the quality of life of those they are caring for at all stages of the disease process. Carers include those paid to care as well as relatives, friends and neighbours who act as informal or unpaid carers.

Demands upon informal carers can be both physical and emotional, often having economic and health consequences for the unpaid caregiver. The demands of the caring role can be so great that it can create high levels of stress in the carer (Gilhooly 1984). Within a framework devised to describe the burden of informal carers, Nolan, Grant and Ellis (1990) also identified loss of social life and loss of the previous relationship with the cared for. It therefore follows that in the case of people with dementia living at home and being supported by family or friends, interventions should not be delivered in isolation from their living situation. Recognition of the needs of informal carers was formally acknowledged through the Carers (Recognition and Services) Act 1995, with the subsequent Carers and Disabled Children Act 2000 enabling the provision of services to carers in their own right.

Interventions with informal carers can take several forms, for example:

- provision of information and advice
- teaching coping and rehabilitative strategies so that the carer is able to facilitate independence in the person they are caring for
- counselling and support
- assessment for, and provision of, assistive devices and adaptations to the home to compensate for diminished capacities in the person being cared for, and to assist the carer.

Those paid to care for people with dementia also face challenges. This is particularly so for those working with people with severe illness. It is important to provide staff with strategies that help them to enable the people they care for, as well as providing a sense of job satisfaction. The engagement of staff is essential to the success of any programme of rehabilitation or care.

It was therefore important to include the evidence regarding interventions with carers within the rubric of research concerned with rehabilitation of people with dementia.

The search strategy

The search strategy had to take account of the nature of the evidence base and the purpose of the search. Issues to be considered included the following:

- Rehabilitation with people with dementia is a previously neglected area of interest for the majority; therefore the evidence base is sparse, less accessible and less robust. However, noteworthy examples of service innovation might be used to inform the practice in the absence of research.

- Interventions are not consistently described as rehabilitation. A number of other key terms were identified as the search proceeded, for example, memory training.

- The purpose of the review was to identify the bodies of evidence that exist and are developing. Therefore, coverage of topics was prioritized over providing a systematic search of available evidence in defined areas. Readers with interest in specific areas are encouraged to undertake further, in-depth, quality reviews.

Results of the search

Taking into account that people with dementia come from a wide range of circumstances, and that carers are frequently involved, the following nine domains that can fall within the rubric of rehabilitation were identified through the search yield:

1.   Assessment of function.

2.   Psychosocial activities.

3.   Psychotherapeutic modalities, for example, reminiscence therapy.

4.   Sensory stimulation, for example, music and Snoezelen.

5.   Interventions to improve functional ability and abilities to undertake activities of daily living.

6.   Interventions to improve memory and cognition.

7.   Self-management.

8.   Technologies to compensate for failing mental and physical capacities.

9.   Interventions to assist both formal (paid) and informal (relatives, friends and neighbours) carers.

What is described below provides some examples of what is available, and gives an indication of how current thinking in this area is progressing. It also demonstrates where further research effort should be directed.

Assessment of function

Even though people with dementia are frequently assessed, this search uncovered only two examples of evidence of assessment as an integral part of the rehabilitation process. Tullis and Nicol (1999) reported the results of a systematic review of the evidence to support functional assessment of older people with dementia. Results confirmed the current lack of evidence to support or refute the undertaking of these assessments.

The Assessment of Process and Motor Skills (AMPS) has been developed primarily for use by occupational therapists. It is an observational assessment used to measure the quality of the individual's performance in activities of daily living (Fisher 1999). It has been used with people with dementia, enabling the therapist to help the individual to adapt their performance. Efficiency, safety and independence are measured in 16 domains. Research into the application and outcomes of AMPS is ongoing.

Psychosocial activities

Studies of psychosocial activities were located within literature concerned with psychology, nursing and occupational therapy. Similar findings were described by all of the reviewed studies. However, interpretations of results differed depending upon the professional orientation of the author. Also, it was evident that authors tended to identify evidence from their own professional group rather than considering the totality of what exists.

A comparatively early study considered that occupation for people with dementia in the form of social and recreational activities could present opportunities for social interaction that might not otherwise exist (Jenkins *et al.* 1977).

Law *et al.* (1999) systematically reviewed published research concerned with activity programmes for older persons with dementia. The aims of the review were to examine the effectiveness of activity programmes with respect to improved participation in self-care, productivity and leisure, and improved performance (physical, affective and cognitive). The review identified 19 relevant studies involving a range of interventions, for example:

- functional rehabilitation in a long term care setting
- programme of occupation in a day centre
- walking and conversation in nursing homes
- self-care, leisure and social activities
- AMPS (assessment of motor and process skills) in a day care unit
- individualized ADL (activities of daily living programmes)
- mental stimulation
- music.

Results found that overall some activity programmes were beneficial. However, the available evidence was weak with more rigorous research being required. When the four most robust studies alone were considered, positive treatment effects were revealed, such as improved well-being, communication, mental status and emotional state. These findings were confirmed by a later systematic review by Marshall and Hutchinson (2001) drawing largely upon the evidence available in the nursing literature.

The body of work in neurophysiology has demonstrated that engagement in activities by older people with dementia can increase engagement with the physical and/or social environment (Camp 2001). The need to carefully adapt activities to limit the adverse effects of cognitive impairment was also noted. Buettner *et al.* (1996) examined the use of therapeutic recreation for older people with dementia resident in long-stay care. Two groups were compared over eight weeks. One received traditional group activities. The second received a new schedule (including activities not previously provided) and a programme incorporating an individual developmental approach to exercise and motor skills. Group comparison found that those who received the new schedule had improved grip strength and flexibility and were less agitated. However, this might have been as much to do with the individual nature of the intervention and the increased involvement of staff as with the nature of the programme.

Perrin and May (2000) suggested that cognitive activities like quizzes and reality orientation are redundant for people with severe dementia. They have promoted the notion of undertaking playful activities with severely impaired individuals. This may include child-like pastimes like playing with dolls and beach balls. Even though this approach is skilled, following training it can be delivered by all grades of staff within a service setting.

Psychotherapeutic modalities

Reminiscence therapy, validation therapy and reality orientation therapies are popular treatment modalities for people with dementia. They have been subjected to more rigorous scrutiny than other forms of intervention. Spector *et al.* (1998a) conducted a review to examine the effectiveness of reminiscence therapy for people with dementia, using the following definition:

> Vocal or silent recall of events in a person's life, either alone, or with another person or group of people. It typically involves group meetings, at least once a week, in which participants are encouraged to talk about past events, often assisted by aids such as photos, music, objects and videos of the past.

The results of the review provided the following tentative implications for practice:

- Reminiscence therapy should be part of a continuous, ongoing programme or incorporated into the daily routine.
- Assessment for inclusion should include psychological as well as cognitive factors.
- It may be more successful in the early stages of dementia.

Spector *et al.* (1998b) also undertook a review of reality orientation. This was identified as:

> A technique to improve the quality of life of confused elderly people…it operates through the presentation of orientation information (eg time, place and person related) which is thought to provide the person with a greater understanding of their surroundings, possibly resulting in an improved sense of control and self esteem.

Results showed that reality orientation is beneficial. However, it is difficult to identify the aspects that provide most benefit, for example, amount and quality of input. The implications for practice were that classroom reality orientation can lead to cognitive and behavioural improvements in the short term, but there is no evidence of long-term benefit, however, improvement might be sustained through an ongoing programme. The main drawback is rigid, inappropriate application.

A study by Metitieri *et al.* (2001) of reality orientation indicated that when it is delivered in the early to middle stages of dementia over an extended period of time it may delay nursing home admission and slow down cognitive decline.

Validation therapy is a third approach often used with older people with dementia. It is defined as:

> A therapy for communicating with old-old people who are diagnosed as having Alzheimer's disease and related dementia. (Neal and Briggs 1999, p.1)

It validates the communication of the person, rather than correcting an erroneous understanding as in reality orientation. Neal and Briggs (1999) conducted a systematic review of validation therapy. It was not possible to draw definitive conclusions about benefit due to lack of evidence. The authors noted that benefit might be derived through the improved attitudes of those providing care.

Sensory stimulation

The effectiveness of music therapy as a treatment modality was explored through a meta analysis of studies (Koger, Chapin and Brotons 1999). The conclusions drawn were that music or music therapy is effective for treating the symptoms of dementia. However, this was based on the findings of some weak studies and, as the authors pointed out, the aspects that result in benefit have not been determined.

Snoezelen was first developed as a treatment modality for people with learning disabilities and has since been used with other client groups with multiple and severe impairments. It involves the use of equipment to stimulate the senses in an attractive, non-demanding manner, thus creating an enjoyable relaxing environment. Van Diepen *et al.* (2002) reported a pilot study to examine the effects of Snoezelen for people with dementia, compared with reminiscence therapy. Results suggested that both treatments can have short-term effects like reduction of agitation, leading to a more relaxed state in some people and increased stimulation for others. Most recently a Cochrane Review to examine the effectiveness of Snoezelen for dementia concluded that the evidence base is as yet insufficient to be able to draw definitive conclusions regarding benefit (Chung *et al.* 2003).

Interventions to improve functional ability and abilities to undertake activities of daily living

The ability to undertake functional tasks and improve daily living skills has been the focus of specialized, hospital-based rehabilitation services for people with physical injury or illness. Physical rehabilitation for people with physical problems as well as dementia has been a neglected dimension.

Huusko *et al.* (2000) evaluated the impact of intensive geriatric rehabilitation for people with dementia who had sustained a hip fracture. The study was a sub analysis of a larger four year study of the effectiveness of rehabilitation for older people with hip fracture. All 238 participants with dementia had been fully mobile prior to injury. Results found that people with hip fracture and mild or moderate dementia can often return to the community. Moreover, the three months post-operative rate of return home for those with mild dementia was as successful as for people with no dementia.

Rydholm Hedman and Grafström (2001) also studied the rehabilitation of older people with dementia and hip fracture through a much smaller study which also involved the next of kin of patients. Results indicated that cognitive function is not the overriding influencing factor, dictating ability to be able to participate in physical rehabilitation such as gait training, and that engagement can be improved through staff support. This study illustrated the underlying complexity underpinning decisions regarding competence to manage rehabilitation. The authors concluded that the ability of the staff to identify and solve problems that can prevent rehabilitation is of vital importance.

In contrast, a randomized controlled trial to examine the benefits of physiotherapy for people with Alzheimer's disease admitted to hospital for respite care showed no statistically significant benefits for participants (Pomeroy *et al.* 1999). The authors questioned whether the positive effects observed through other studies were due to the overall extent of activity being undertaken rather than that limited to specific rehabilitative interventions.

Interventions to improve memory and cognition

Katz (1994) identified two main approaches towards the treatment of cognitive deficit. The remedial approach presumes that the brain has the potential to recover, and therefore that cognitive impairments can be treated directly. Alternatively, the functional approach is that the brain has limited potential to recover and that training and practice are required together with the adaptation of tasks and environments. The remedial approach has exclusively been promoted with people with dementia, but this is now being challenged. There is an ongoing body of work, largely by psychologists, exploring the potential of memory training for people with mild to moderate dementia. Techniques under examination embrace the investigation of traditional such as memory aids as well as those using new forms of technology.

The Cochrane database of systematic reviews has established the Cochrane Dementia and Cognitive Improvement Group. This group has devised a review protocol to examine cognitive rehabilitation interventions to improve memory function in early stage Alzheimer's disease and vascular dementia (Clare *et al.* 2001). The definition of cognitive rehabilitation being used by the group includes:

- helping people to utilize their remaining memory most effectively
- compensating for difficulties, for example, through the use of memory aids
- environmental adjustments so that demands on memory are reduced.

De Vreese *et al.* (2001) conducted a rigorous overview of memory rehabilitation in dementia, drawing upon the existing evidence. The review was underpinned by the notion that the introduction of acetylcholinersterase inhibitors (so called anti dementia drugs), which have been shown to temporarily allay cognitive decline in people with dementia, opens up new treatment possibilities. Results suggested that some people with Alzheimer's disease can benefit from memory rehabilitation, but more research is required. Additionally they pointed out that informal and/or paid carers are necessary to ensure that interventions are undertaken correctly.

Work is being undertaken to explore the potential of computerized packages for rehabilitation. Schreiber *et al.* (1999) described the development and testing of a computerized memory training programme for people with mild to moderate dementia. The results of this research (which at the time of writing was in its early stages of development) indicated the value of pursuing this work further. Lekeu *et al.* (2002) reported a study to look at the potential of the mobile phone for people with early Alzheimer's disease. They trained two people to use the phone using specific techniques. The subjects demonstrated different learning abilities, but at the end of training both were able to make correct calls. The authors suggested that this demonstrated relatively preserved procedural memory, making it possible to learn and re-teach actions that are useful in everyday life. However, it would be important to assess abilities at frequent intervals.

More traditional forms of intervention are also under scrutiny. Werner (2000) conducted a small scale year-long evaluation of a memory club for people with mild cognitive impairment. This group offered social activities as well as memory training activities. Results of analysis of the abilities of 19 people who remained in the programme showed that while a statistically significant decrease was observed in overall cognitive function, memory function was at least maintained, and in some cases improved. This was partly attributed to the greater awareness that participants had of their memory problems as well as the development of strategies for self-management.

Hoerster, Hickey and Bourgeois (2001) explored the use of personalized memory books (prepared with the help of friends and relations) on nursing home residents with dementia. This small scale study only involved four older women, all with tested cognitive abilities sufficient for reading. Four nursing assistants were recruited to the study to work with each of the women. Results found that all four women improved to some extent in their ability to engage in verbal and non-verbal communication when using their memory aid. The nursing assistants were observed to change their approach so that conversation focused upon the residents, with subsequent improvement in communication. The authors suggested that the observed benefits of this fairly simple procedure warrant further investigation.

Interesting possibilities offered by Montessori methods of education are being explored. Orsulic-Jeras and colleagues (2000) experimented with the use of activities for people in long-term care based upon Montessori principles. This method of learning, originally developed for use with nursery children, comprises task breakdown, guided repetition and progressive upgrading of activities. Results showed that the Montessori activities were associated with significant increase in engagement and pleasure and less negative behaviours. The authors postulated that this was due to the underlying use of rehabilitative principles.

Self-management

Methods of self-management of chronic illnesses are well described in relation to illnesses like arthritis and manic depressive psychosis, and are a key element of current government policy as described through the expert patient initiative (DH 2001c). To date, possibilities for people with dementia tend to have been set aside. However, two studies were located during the review that considered self-management as part of packages of interventions.

Work by Bach et al. (1995) compared two occupational therapy intervention strategies with long-term patients with mild to moderate dementia. One group received a functional rehabilitation programme including occupational therapy, physiotherapy and speech therapy. The second group received this programme as well as additional group occupational therapy twice a week, incorporating memory training, occupations to improve sensorimotor functions and activities to promote self management. After 24 weeks all 44 participants showed overall improvement in abilities but the group allocated to extra occupational therapy showed significantly greater abilities in cognitive performance, a decrease in symptoms and improved subjective well-being. The authors postulated that this difference might have been due to the stimulation of latent resources of cognition and socialization, resulting in improved life quality, but also stressed the importance of not demanding too much or building false expectations of recovery.

Romero and Wenz (2001) reported the evaluation of a programme that aimed to prepare people with dementia and their carers for life with a progressive, degenerative disease. The self-management aspect of the programme included maintenance of a sense of personal identity through activities (like those discussed in previous sections of this chapter), the provision of psychotherapeutic support to give people an understanding of their illness and how to manage it, and engagement in everyday activities. Additionally, family carers were helped to understand the reasons for the changed behaviour of the person they cared for and how to maintain communication. Statistical analysis showed that the level of depression and other psychiatric symptoms experienced by participants decreased and there was some improvement in social behaviour. Caregivers also reported an improvement in their mood. The authors stressed the need for controlled studies to support these results.

Technologies to compensate for failing mental and physical capacities

The findings of the review revealed a range of services to compensate for diminishing capacities and promote independence. These services are not rehabilitative in themselves and new developments are leading to blurring of their specific functions. Woolham and Frisby (2002) identified three categories of technology that can be placed in an existing property to monitor a person and alert assistance if indicated:

1. Stand alone technologies that do not link into other systems.

2. Technologies based on community alarms, and can include smoke and gas detectors.

3. SMART systems that filter information from a range of sensors linked to a computer system installed in the user's home.

It should be noted that these technologies are not specific to people with dementia, though the particular benefits of these technologies for people with cognitive decline are now being realized. This is reflected in the following literature.

COMMUNITY EQUIPMENT/ ASSISTIVE TECHNOLOGY

Current interpretations of assistive technology embrace simple items, like walking sticks and bath seats, and technological developments, like devices to shut off gas appliances. Studies of the use of assistive technology by people with cognitive impairment (Mann *et al.* 1992, 1996, quoted in Yang *et al.* 1997) have found that most device use is focused upon enabling physical rather than cognitive abilities, with the majority of equipment being used to facilitate safety. Use of devices to assist cognition declined over time, but equipment usage to help care givers with activities of daily living increased.

ENVIRONMENTAL PROMPTS OR CONTROLS

Environmental control systems (ECS) enable a person to have control over their environment through the use of technology. Vincent, Drouin and Routhier (1999) conducted five case studies with different types of user to examine the success of ECS in increasing independence of the person and reducing the burden upon their carer. The study found that while the systems reduced the dependency of the individuals, caregiver burden remained high. The stress upon carers was reduced when the system worked, but increased when it failed. It also did not reduce the burden associated with activities such as dressing, shopping, transport and budgeting.

Experiments are taking place to develop and test devices that are able to prompt people with dementia to undertake appropriate activities of daily living, and thus retain their independence and dignity. Mihailidis, Fernie and Cleghorn (2000) developed a prototype computerized device to prompt an individual to undertake the sequence of actions required to wash their hands. Use of the device prompted the activity and reduced caregiver intervention. This is an area where far more experimentation is required. The press reported a similar approach in June 2003 (BBC News 2003). A robot linked to a remote computer has been developed in North America. The reported trial of the device within a care home is able to link health care professionals with the person with dementia, who is able to undertake a conversation with the screen. This initial work showed that the subjects had no problems communicating with the device.

Interventions to assist both formal (paid) and informal (relatives, friends and neighbours) carers

Intervention with carers can take several forms, including the provision of information, counselling, education and training; the use of technology to support carers; and teaching coping and rehabilitative strategies so that the carer is able to manage the needs of the person they are caring for more effectively.

PROVISION OF INFORMATION, COUNSELLING, EDUCATION AND TRAINING

Mitchell (2000) described the initiation and evaluation of a four-week stress management programme for carers in the health education room of a local hospital. Carers were expected to transport themselves to the group, with care for the person they cared for being made available. The tentative results of this small scale study were that carer awareness was improved and there was a decrease in some of the aspects of burden they experienced at the time.

Carers may wish to take the opportunity to learn enabling skills to assist the person they care for. Respite care can be used to provide rehabilitative interventions to both carer and their cared for, as a means of improving quality of life

(Nolan and Grant 1993). Brodaty, Gresham and Luscombe (1997) reported the results of a prospective randomized controlled trial of a training programme for co-resident informal carers of people under 80 years of age with mild to moderate dementia. Ninety-six people with dementia and their carers participated in the trial, which commenced in 1989. An already established ten-day memory retraining and activity programme was delivered to people with dementia. Additionally, carers were randomized to receive intensive residential training immediately. Taking into account the fact that the numbers in each group were not adequate to allow firm conclusions to be drawn from statistical analysis, the eight-year survival analysis indicated that the people whose caregivers received training stayed at home longer rather than being admitted to institutional care, and tended to live longer. A further study by Brodaty, Green and Koschera (2003) involved a meta analysis of 30 studies of interventions with carers of people with dementia. The conclusions drawn from this synthesis were that some interventions could reduce stress experienced by carers and help them to continue caring for longer. Those interventions that involve the person with dementia and their families on an intensive basis are more likely to be successful. The inadequacy of the current evidence base was also raised.

The complexity of undertaking research into interventions for people with dementia and their carers is illustrated through the work of Gitlin *et al.* (2001). They conducted a randomized controlled trial to look at the short-term effects of occupational therapy interventions in the homes upon co-resident carers of people with dementia. Two hundred volunteer families of people with dementia were recruited and randomized to an intervention or control group. Those receiving the intervention had five 90-minute home visits over a three-month period by an occupational therapist who worked to a protocol devised and evaluated previously by the authors (Gitlin *et al.* 1999 reported in Gitlin *et al.* 2001). This entailed educating carers about the impact of the environment on behaviours of people with dementia and suggesting strategies like removing clutter, breaking down tasks into simple commands and involving other family members and social support in caring tasks. The results indicated that the intervention promoted the continued independence of the people with dementia. It also enabled female carers to cope, and reduced distress in spouse carers. The authors concluded that there is a need to develop different strategies for different types of carer, as the effect of the intervention did not have the same impact on male as on female carers. The same group of researchers has been working on the development of a systematic approach to caregiver education through the development of a task management strategy index for carers (TMSI) (Gitlin *et al.* 2002). Initial testing of the instrument showed that educating informal carers correlated highly with greater use of specific coping strategies.

USE OF TECHNOLOGY TO SUPPORT CARERS

A number of projects have been reported to examine the potential of technology in assisting and supporting carers of older people (not exclusively with dementia). A Europe-wide project to explore the use of technology to support carers' needs for information, education and support was reported by Hanson and Clarke (2000). Despite an approach being made to 12 family carers, only 3 agreed to participate in user trials of the technology. The researchers attributed the low response to invitations to participate in the project to the length of time most had been caring. User evaluation of the technology developed during this project was reported by Chambers and Connor (2002). Most of the participants considered it to be helpful and were also able to suggest modifications to the devices. Some carers felt that they did not have adequate time to devote to the project, particularly where their caring situation demanded a lot of time.

The authors raised the importance of involving users carefully in design issues as well as subsequent evaluation. Woolham and Frisby (2002) explored whether technology could be used to reduce the stress experienced by carers of older people with dementia, and to delay admission to residential care. Devices were linked to community alarms, so that the alarm was activated when the older person was at risk. The study concluded that the successful use of technology in this way requires a robust service infrastructure including mechanisms for support and review.

TRAINING CARE STAFF TO ENABLE

The need for education for care staff was underscored by research undertaken in a day care setting for people with Alzheimer's disease (Hasselkus 1992). The research included participant observation by the author, interviews with the three staff and a document analysis. Results found that the main aim of the setting was to prevent the attendees harming themselves. Emphasis was placed upon a calming environment and making sure that any trouble was caught early. Only when safety was ensured were other aims like enjoyment and individualized care met. It was also noted that the main emphasis of care was engagement in group activities. The need to identify the sources of satisfaction for staff working with this highly disabled group was raised.

A comprehensive systematic review of the literature on the primary management of dementia is contained within the Cochrane Library (North of England Evidence Based Guideline Development Project 1998). One of the conclusions drawn from the review was that skills training for people with dementia in residential care might lead to an improvement in personal care skills. However, this would require the role of residential care staff to adapt to that of enabling.

Limitations of the current evidence base

This review confirmed the research neglect of many dimensions that can be included within a construct of rehabilitation for people with dementia. Much of the research that exists is small scale, and therefore must therefore be treated with caution, particularly in the case of quantitative projects. This observation is confirmed by Marshall and Hutchinson (2001). Their systematic review drew attention to the limitations of projects involving small numbers of subjects and conducted using weak methodology, with resulting unsubstantiated conclusions. The exception to this is the more robust work of Huusko and colleagues (2000) where a greater number of subjects enabled more robust conclusions to be drawn regarding the importance of an inclusive approach towards medical rehabilitation. A further observation by Marshall and Hutchinson (2001) was that little attention had been given to research that is home rather than institutionally based. The exception to this is the ongoing work reported by Gitlin and others in North America.

A more extensive body of evidence exists in the psychology literature with respect to memory training and self maintenance; only a few examples have been quoted here. However, at present this work is difficult to access. Furthermore, the jump from empirical study by psychologists and other scientists to practical applications in the home, ward or residential care setting has yet to be made.

It is evident that there is an urgent need for substantial funded projects to test the population benefit of different aspects of rehabilitation with people with dementia. There is also a need for more rigorous qualitative studies so that our understanding of the impact of rehabilitation upon different individuals with dementia, and their carers, is improved. Given that it will take time to further develop the evidence base, in the meantime what exists already must be translated into formats that make it accessible, useful and informative.

Creating an evidence-based construct of rehabilitation for people with dementia

The commonly held view that people with dementia cannot learn new skills and, therefore, any intervention is at best going to fail and at worst have an adverse effect upon the person and their carer is being challenged. (Camp 2001) proposed that this negative attitude has led to a lack of training in appropriate interventions for those working with people with dementia, resulting in 'self-fulfilling prophecies' whereby the results of treatment are not maintained because of no interventions or inadequate interventions due to lack of skill on the part of the caregiver. Other research undertaken by occupational therapists has indicated that people with Alzheimer's disease are aware of their disabilities, at least in the early to mid stages of the illness, and are able to adopt self-management strategies (Nygard and Ohman 2002).

This review has clearly demonstrated the value of the creation of a construct of rehabilitation that is *specific to the needs of people with dementia.* This construct needs to take into account quality of life in its widest sense, and be sufficiently flexible. It has also confirmed the importance of adopting strategies appropriate to the level of impairment. The evidence base suggests that for those people with mild to moderate difficulties, there may well be a benefit in adopting a rehabilitative approach grounded in restoration of physical function and maintenance of cognitive abilities. In contrast, for those with severe difficulties, this becomes redundant, with the requirements moving towards providing a safe environment that promotes the quality of life of the individual and maintains their sense of person, both for themselves and the people caring for them. The need for approaches that are underpinned by assessment of need, enabling the construction of an individualized, person-centred approach is evident. The evidence base also confirms that carer involvement is crucial throughout.

Conclusions

Rehabilitation for people with dementia is not a new concept. Some practitioners have been working within rehabilitative principles for many years. What is different is the acknowledgement of the benefits that rehabilitation can bring to a group previously considered to be incapable of using rehabilitation successfully. Translation of rehabilitation policy into action is taking place at a rapid rate. This review has confirmed that people with dementia can benefit from hospital led rehabilitation as well as from rehabilitation delivered under the auspices of social care.

We need to ensure that people with dementia are included in new ways of thinking and consequent service developments rather than being marginalized. The evidence and knowledge that already exists needs translating into a practice framework and disseminating as a matter of urgency. Furthermore, the evidence and knowledge base that is at present 'owned' by researchers from specific professions needs to be shared so that multidisciplinary teams can readily access information regarding new and developing areas of practice. Finally, this review has confirmed the importance of adopting an open mind regarding what might be achieved with people with a diagnosis of dementia, taking into account the new avenues that technology and alternative forms of provision are opening up.

References

Allan, K. (2001) *Communication and Consultation: Exploring Ways for Staff to Involve People with Dementia in Developing Services.* York: Policy Press and Joseph Rowntree Foundation.

Bach, D., Bach, M., Böhmer, F., Frühwald, T. and Grilic, B. (1995) 'Reactivating occupational therapy: a method to improve cognitive performance in geriatric patients.' *Age and Ageing 24*, 3, 222–226.

BBC News (June 2003) 'Robot helps dementia patients.' news.bbc.co.uk/1/hi/health/2830533.stm

Benson, S. (ed) (2000) 'Creative approaches to individualised care for people with dementia.' *Journal of Dementia Care*, person centred series. Also available from Bradford Dementia Group: www.brad.ac.uk/acad/health/bdg

Brodaty, H., Gresham, M. and Luscombe, G. (1997) 'The Prince Henry Hospital Dementia Caregivers programme.' *International Journal of Geriatric Psychiatry 12*, 2, 183–192.

Brodaty, H., Green, A. and Koschera, A. (2003) 'Meta analysis of pychosocial interventions for caregivers of people with dementia.' *Journal of the American Geriatrics Society 51*, 5, 657–664.

Buettner, L.L., Lundegren, H., Lago, D., Farrell, P. and Smith, R. (1996) 'Therapeutic recreation as an intervention for persons with dementia and agitation: An efficacy study.' *American Journal of Alzheimer's Disease* Sept/ Oct 1996, 4–10.

Camp, C.J. (2001) 'From efficacy to effectiveness to diffusion. Making the transitions in dementia intervention research.' *Neuropsychological Rehabilitation 11*, 3/4, 496–517.

Carers (Recognition and Services) Act 1995. London: HMSO.

Carers and Disabled Children Act 2000. London: HMSO.

Chambers, M. and Connor, S.L. (2002) 'User friendly technology to help family carers cope.' *Journal of Advanced Nursing 40*, 5, 568–577.

Chung, J.C.C., Lai, C.K.Y., Chung, P.M.B. and French, H.P. (2003) 'Snoezelen for dementia (Cochrane Review).' *The Cochrane Library* Issue 1, Oxford: update software.

Clare, L., Woods, R.T., Moniz Cook, E.D., Orrell, M. and Spector, A. (2001) 'Cognitive rehabilitation interventions to improve memory functioning in early-stage Alzheimer's disease and vascular dementia (protocol for a Cochrane Review).' *The Cochrane Library* Issue 2, 2001.

Department of Health (2000) *The NHS Plan.* London: DH.

Department of Health (2001a) *The National Service Framework for Older People.* London: DH.

Department of Health (2001b) *Intermediate Care.* HSC 2001/01:LAC. London: DH.

Department of Health (2001c) *The Expert Patient: A New Approach to Chronic Disease Management for the 21st Century.* London: DH.

De Vreese, L.P., Neri, M., Fioravanti, M., Belloi, L. and Zanetti, O. (2001) 'Memory rehabilitation in Alzheimer's disease: a review of progress.' *International Journal of Geriatric Psychiatry 16*, 794–809.

Fisher, A.G. (1999) *Assessment of Motor and Process Skills* (3rd edn). Fort Collins, CO: Three Star Press. colostate.edu/programs/AMPS

Gilhooly, M.L. (1984) 'The impact of caring on care-givers: factors associated with the psychological well-being of people supporting a demented relative in the community.' *British Journal of Medical Psychology 57*, 35–44.

Gitlin, L.N., Corcoran, M., Winter, L., Boyce, A. and Hauck, W.W. (2001) 'A randomised controlled trial of a home environmental intervention: Effect on efficacy and upset in caregivers and on daily function of persons with dementia.' *The Gerontologist 42*, 1, 4–14.

Gitlin, L.N., Winter, L., Dennis, M.P., Corcoran, M., Schinfield, S. and Hauck, W.W. (2002) 'Strategies used by families to simplify tasks for individuals with Alzheimer's disease and related disorders: Pyschometric analysis of the Task Management Strategy Index.' *The Gerontologist 42*, 1, 61–69.

Hanson, E.J. and Clarke, A. (2000) 'The role of telematics in assisting family carers and frail older people at home.' *Health and Social Care in the Community 8*, 2, 129–137.

Hasselkus, B.R. (1992) 'The meaning of activity: Day care for persons with Alzheimer's disease.' *American Journal of Occupational Therapy 46*, 3, 199–206.

Hoerster, L., Hickey, E.M. and Bourgeois, M.S. (2001) 'Effects of memory aids on conversations between nursing home residents with dementia and nursing assistants.' *Neuropsychological Rehabilitation 11*, 3–4, 399–427.

Huusko, T.M., Karppi, P., Avikainen, V., Kautiainen, H. and Sulkava, R. (2000) 'Randomised, clinically controlled trial of intensive geriatric rehabilitation in patients with hip fracture: Subgroup analysis of patients with dementia.' *British Medical Journal 321*, 1107–1111.

Jenkins, J., Felce, D., Lunt, B. and Powell, L. (1977) 'Increasing engagement in activity of residents in old people's homes by providing recreational materials.' *Behaviour Therapy Research 15*, 429–434.

Katz, N. (1994) 'Cognitive rehabilitation: models for intervention and research on cognition in occupational therapy.' *Occupational Therapy International 1*, 49–63.

Kitwood, T. (1993) 'Towards a theory of dementia care: The interpersonal process.' *Ageing and Society 13*, 51–67.

Kitwood, T. (1997) *Dementia Reconsidered*. Buckingham: Open University Press.

Koger, S., Chapin, K. and Brotons, M. (1999) 'Is music therapy an effective intervention for dementia: A meta-analytic review of the literature.' *Journal of Music Therapy 36*, 1, 2–15.

Law, M., Stewart, D., Letts, L., Pollock, N., Westmorland, M., Bosch, J. and Philpot, A. (1999) *Effectiveness of Activity Programmes for Older Persons with Dementia: A Critical Review of the Evidence*. McMaster University, Hamilton Ontario Occupational Therapy Evidence-Based Practice Research Group.

Lekeu, F., Wojtasik, V., Van der Linden, M. and Salmon, E. (2002) 'Training early Alzheimer patients to use a mobile phone.' *Acta Neurologica Belgica 102*, 3, 114–121.

Marshall, M.J. and Hutchinson, S.A. (2001) 'A critique of research on the use of activities with persons with Alzheimer's disease: A systematic literature review.' *Journal of Advanced Nursing 35*, 4, 488–496.

Metitieri, T., Zanetti, O., Geroldi, C., Frisoni, G.B., De Leo, D., Dello Bueno, M., Bianchetti, A. and Trabucchi, M. (2001) 'Reality orientation therapy to delay outcomes of progression in patients with dementia. A retrospective study.' *Clinical Rehabilitation 15*, 471–478.

Mihailidis, A., Fernie, G.R. and Cleghorn, W.L. (2000) 'The development of a computerised cueing device to help people with dementia to be more independent.' *Technology and Disability 13*, 23–40.

Mitchell, E. (2000) 'Managing carer stress: An evaluation of a stress management programme for carers of people with dementia.' *British Journal of Occupational Therapy 63*, 4, 179–183.

Mountain, G. (2001) 'Social rehabilitation: Concepts, evidence and practice.' *Managing Community Care 9*, 2, 8–15.

Neal, M. and Briggs, M. (1999) 'Validation therapy for dementia (Cochrane Review).' *The Cochrane Library* Issue 1, 2000 Oxford: Update Software.

Nolan, M. and Grant, G. (1993) 'Service evaluation: time to open both eyes.' *Journal of Advanced Nursing 18*, 1434–1442.

Nolan, M.R., Grant, G. and Ellis, N.C. (1990) 'Stress is in the eye of the beholder: Reconceptualising the measurement of carer burden.' *Journal of Advanced Nursing 15*, 544–555.

North of England Evidence Based Guideline Development Project (1998) *Evidence Based Clinical Guideline: The Primary Care Management of Dementia.* University of Newcastle upon Tyne: Department of Primary Care.

Nuffield Institute for Health (2002) *Exclusivity or Inclusion? Meeting Mental Health Needs in Intermediate Care.* Leeds: Nuffield Institute for Health with the Joseph Rowntree Foundation.

Nygard, L. and Ohman, A. (2002) 'Managing changes in everyday occupations: The experience of persons with Alzheimer's disease.' *Occupational Therapy Journal of Research 22*, 4, 70–81.

Orsulic-Jeras, S., Schneider, N.M. and Camp, C.J. (2000) 'Special feature: Montessori-based activities for long term care residents with dementia.' *Topics in Geriatric Rehabilitation 16*, 1, 78–91.

Perrin, T. (1997) 'Occupational needs in severe dementia: A descriptive study.' *Journal of Advanced Nursing 25*, 934–941.

Perrin, T. and May, H. (2000) *Wellbeing in Dementia: An Occupational Approach for Therapists and Carers.* London: Churchill Livingstone.

Pomeroy, V.M., Warren, C.M., Honeycombe, C., Briggs, R.S.J., Wilkinson, D.G., Pickering, R.M. and Steiner, A. (1999) 'Mobility and dementia: Is physiotherapy treatment during respite care effective?' *International Journal of Geriatric Psychiatry 14*, 389–397.

Robinson, J. and Batstone, G. (1996) *Rehabilitation: A Development Challenge.* London: King's Fund.

Romero, B. and Wenz, M. (2001) 'Self maintenance therapy in Alzheimer's disease.' *Neuropsychological Rehabilitation 11*, 3–4, 335–355.

Rydholm Hedman, A.-M. and Grafström, M. (2001) 'Conditions for rehabilitation of older patients with dementia and hip fracture – the perspective of their next of kin.' *Scandinavian Journal of Caring Services 15*, 2, 151–158.

Schreiber, M., Schweizer, A., Lutz, K., Kalverham, K.T. and Lutz, J. (1999) 'Potential of an interactive computer-based training in the rehabilitation of dementia: An initial study.' *Neuropsychological Rehabilitation 9*, 2, 155–167.

Spector, A., Orrell, M., Davies, S. and Woods, R.T. (1998a) 'Reminiscence therapy for dementia (Cochrane Review).' *The Cochrane Library Issue 1*, 2000, Oxford: Update Software.

Spector, A., Orrell, M., Davies, S. and Woods, R.T. (1998b) 'Reality orientation for dementia (Cochrane Review).' *The Cochrane Library Issue 1*, 2000, Oxford: Update Software.

Tullis, A. and Nicol, M. (1999) 'A systematic review of the evidence for the value of functional assessments of older people with dementia.' *British Journal of Occupational Therapy 62*, 12, 554–563.

Van Diepen, E., Baillon, S., Redman, J., Rooke, N., Spencer, D.A. and Prettyman, R. (2002) 'A pilot study of the physiological and behavioural effects of Snoezelen in dementia.' *British Journal of Occupational Therapy 65*, 2, 61–66.

Vincent, C., Drouin, G. and Routhier, F. (1999) *Environmental Control Systems for Disabled and Older Adults: A Challenge on the Threshold of a New Millennium.* Germany, Proceeding of the AAATE Conference 1999.

Werner, P. (2000) 'Assessing the effectiveness of a memory club for elderly persons suffering from mild cognitive impairment.' *Clinical Gerontologist 22*, 1, 3–14.

Wey, S. (2002) 'Intensive home-based rehabilitation.' *Journal of Dementia Care 10*, 3, 28–31.

Woolham, J. and Frisby, B. (2002) 'Building a local infrastructure that supports the use of assistive technology in the care of people with dementia.' *Research, Policy and Planning 20*, 1, 11–24.

World Health Organization (2001) *International Classification of Functioning, Disability and Health (ICF).* Geneva: WHO.

Yang, J.-J., Mann, W.C., Nochajski, S. and Tomita, M.R. (1997) 'Use of assistive devices among elders with cognitive impairment: A follow up study.' *Topics in Geriatric Rehabilitation 13*, 2, 13–21.

PART TWO

Perspectives of People with Dementia and their Carers

CHAPTER 6

Rehabilitation: A Carer's Perspective

Susan Fleming

Part of my work, as a support worker for people with dementia and their families, involves helping them to negotiate the health and welfare systems. This frequently involves visiting them when they are in acute hospital wards, and helping carers in their attempts to talk to staff. It concerns me that dementia is frequently not recognized or recorded, so really unhelpful decisions are made. I am a nurse so I am well able to understand the world of NHS wards and to stand up for and with my clients, but it should not be like this. The whole system should recognize the needs of people with dementia and should be geared up to involve their relatives in their care.

All my skills were needed when my father needed surgery. He is a younger person with dementia, and the whole process of diagnosis took months with little in the way of support for him or for us. I had to push really hard to get help for my mother who was struggling to provide 24-hour care. I got a day a week at a day hospital to give her a break but nothing would have happened if I had not pushed for it.

Some months ago my mother found a lump in his chest when she was helping him to wash. He complained of pain too. It took a year to get seen at the hospital. Once seen they moved swiftly to arrange for surgery. He had to go for half a day pre-op, which tired him out, as did the subsequent additional visit for a lung check. Fortunately I was able to drive him and my mother to these appointments. Two weeks later we got an appointment for the actual operation. He was to go in on Monday morning and to have the operation on Tuesday with a further five days in hospital to drain the wound. We sat all day until 5.00 in the hospital waiting room, only to find there was no bed. He was very restless and anxious. This happened again the following Monday. On the third Monday my mother broke down in tears as we sat waiting and we decided that he needed to be at home and to return on Tuesday. This time he got the operation.

At teatime when I went to see him he was up and about. He had apparently pulled out the drainage tubes within five minutes. He was very restless and uncomfortable. We got a phone call on Wednesday saying that they could no longer cope with him and he was to be discharged home. We picked him up at the hospital. There was no follow up at all of any sort. He was exhausted and disorientated for several days when he got home, although he was very glad to be there. It was impossible to know if he was in pain and he was not eating or drinking at all. My mother did not want to call the GP. We persuaded her that this would be necessary if he continued not to eat or drink. Fortunately he settled by Thursday. In retrospect we really wondered whether the operation could not have been done on a one-day basis with lots of home nursing. It had been a real trauma for him and for us.

It became clear to us that the planning of his care was not done with his dementia in mind. I had to continually tell doctors and nurses about it. I cannot imagine how families cope when they are not articulate nurses as we are. We are able to be with our parents in situations like this; but what about a spouse who is older and frail herself or people who are on their own. At times like this people with dementia need familiar people around who provide continuity.

CHAPTER 7

Tedious No More!

Morris Friedell

The caregivers are doing their darndest – they want to be like any other people, and they deserve their moments, their times – their times away from us, because it can be very tedious. We can be very tedious. I can be very tedious, and I'm aware of that. (Henderson 1998, p.82)

Introduction

Unfortunately Cary's lament is not merely a figment of his low self-esteem. Cohen and Eisdorfer, in their authoritative *The Loss of Self* (2001, p.96), go so far as to declare to caregivers: 'Regardless of your personality, professional training, or background, it is hard to be close to the patient for long periods without feeling upset or uncomfortable.' The impact of this repulsive pronouncement becomes evident if we substitute physical disability for mental: 'Regardless of your personality, professional training, or background, it is hard to be close to a person in a wheelchair for long periods without feeling upset or uncomfortable.' To participate pleasantly or productively in social interaction is a major challenge for us PWiDs (persons with dementia).

We're not quite social 'lepers'. Not being wrapped up in our own important thoughts, we can often tune into others' feelings and be warmly responsive to them. TABs (temporarily able-brained persons) enjoy this, and we can be glad to give them a few pleasant moments. But then we must be wary that they don't patronize us.

I am not so sure I would hope for a world without dementia, for in a world without dementia we would be without the ones we love who have taught us that remembering and planning and naming and knowing are not the key activities of human life, but rather that feeling and being and touching and singing have enormous riches and depths that we are often too busy to relish in our race to rationality. (Killick and Allan 2001, p.62)

Men used to often talk this way about women, and failed to understand why the women were not grateful.

Carole Mulliken, a PWiD leader of DASNI (Dementia Advocacy and Support Network International, www.dasninternational.org), summed up as follows the social position dementia has thrust us into: 'a pet, a mortgage, and yesterday's laundry'. No wonder we tend to withdraw and isolate ourselves. Diagnosed with early Alzheimer's disease (AD) in 1998, I mostly live in a social cocoon, interacting with my wife (who is disabled like myself), an old friend and a paid therapist. When I venture out, it is usually on the Internet, not in so-called real time. I don't want to be tedious, I don't want to be pitied, and I don't want to be patronized.

But is it a cocoon I live in – or a ghetto? One of the lessons of the Holocaust is to resist ghettoization. 'Never again!' was an impetus for the Universal Declaration of Human Rights. Its article 27 declares: 'Everyone has the right freely to participate in the cultural life of the community.' In line with this we have women's 'take back the night' campaigns, wheelchair-accessibility, TV programmes with sign-language. It is time for the cognitively impaired to cast off their shame, come out of the closet and fight for their dignity. If not now, when?

This chapter develops some ideas that might help me and might help others in similar situations. The resultant successes and failures will be the subject of a future article.

Concepts

Four years ago I wrote 'Potential for Rehabilitation in Alzheimer's Disease' (Friedell 2000) where I proposed that the qualitative symptoms of mild to moderate AD – disorientation, gross forgetfulness and loss of abstraction and judgment – are susceptible to the rehabilitative interventions used for traumatic brain injury. I have applied these methods to myself and have reduced my Clinical Dementia Rating (CDR) from 1 in 1999 to 0 in 2002 despite MRI evidence of disease progression (but there's no way to predict how long I've got). A basic rehabilitative concept is to relearn activities using a greater number of easier steps, i.e. more slowly.[1] Unfortunately, in daily social life slowness causes problems.

Mitchell and Jonas-Simpson (2003) interviewed persons diagnosed with early-onset dementia and compiled an excellent summary of their experience. They write of 'Slowing Rhythms':

This theme emerged from persons' descriptions of experiencing faster rhythms around them like the world swirling about, while at the same time sensing one's personal rhythms as slower paced. For some it was not until they were…in groups or in situations outside their familiar settings that they realized how slow they had become. Others described watching themselves in a distant way, as if seeing themselves in a movie or through a window. Persons offered examples such as no longer having a quick wit or spontaneous joke… Some persons described feeling frustrated and overwhelmed by the noises and chatter of a fast-paced world…

It is tempting for PWiDs to cope by acting like 'shells': participating appropriately but passively, reactively or superficially. For, as far as I know, we can't recover the processing speed that would allow us to really regain normalcy. Fortunately, normalcy is not important for its own sake. Normal people want, for example, to be somebody or to have fun, not just to be normal. Normalcy is, as it were, a platform for life rather than life itself. So maybe substitutes can be fashioned. 'Why be normal?' says a humorous lapel-button.

What, then, is to be done? I have found some well-reputed self-help books which advocate using 'baby steps' as part of a program to improve one's position in life and I will combine their ideas. Their areas of concern often seem far removed from our topic but nevertheless they offer intriguing possibilities. Of particular interest are Sinetar's *Do What You Love, the Money will Follow* (1987) and Davis' *The Divorce Remedy* (2002). They are written for people who find themselves enmeshed in complex situations (in the domains of work and love, respectively) where their behavior is incongruent with their inner being. Baby steps, requiring minimal cognitive resources, can be part of a program of self-change which recruits support from the environment.

Perhaps my ultimate inspiration comes from the Tao Te Ching, the ancient classic on winning through weakness: 'A journey of a thousand miles begins with a single step.'

Program

Here is an overview of my six steps – references for them are at the end of the chapter.[2] (Those familiar with the steps of Alcoholics Anonymous will note a vague resemblance.)

The first step, *self-awareness*, is to 'clear a space', somewhat detaching yourself from the ongoing situation, so it can be seen in perspective and worked with creatively. This means putting less energy into doing what you have been doing, and coping with the feelings that may then arise, i.e. to withdraw somewhat, if you are not already withdrawn. Rather than ignoring the current reality of the difficult situation or blindly attacking it, it is necessary to desire change but accept your powerlessness to make rapid changes.

Second, *self-reflection*: in the space in your life cleared by the first step, get in touch with what you really value, who you really are, what you really want, and your reasons for hope. What story arises from your memories, your dreams, your vision?

Third, *self-determination*: energize your vision by committing to work toward it every day. Record your work in a journal.

Fourth, *self-appreciation*: at first in small, safe, symbolic ways, express and celebrate who you are. This is primarily a matter between you and yourself.

Fifth, *self-expression*: start taking baby steps toward your dream of expressing your revitalized self in social interaction and being 'tedious no more!' And (where appropriate) tell others about this project, in a manner that orients them to your self and your vision rather than demands their support. Act as if you expect their respect but not agreement. And look for friends who do support your quest.

Sixth, *self-acceptance*: let the dust settle, relax and be centred before returning to step one and beginning another cycle.

Self-expression

Each step is more difficult than it looks, but it is only the fifth step that poses particular difficulties for persons with mild dementia, since it is the only one focused on real-time performance. Thaddeus M. Rauschi's excellent *A View from Within* (2001) clearly illustrates this. Dr Rauschi exhibits an emotional intelligence and spirituality which gives him high marks on the qualities required by steps 1, 2, 3 and 6. As for step 4, he writes:

> Very often I feel so normal, especially when I have been working alone on a project or working at writing (this book for example) at my own pace ... While I take a morning shower (it has always been my 'think tank') and have these wonderful creative ideas and plans, I feel I am so much myself... (p.28)

But alas, when he goes out into society (step 5):

> I can't get the words to participate spontaneously in the interaction, or at least participate well. I can't think fast enough to follow the ideas... (p.75)

He has found some ways to cope, and I hope the framework presented here could help make them more systematic and effective.

Jeanne L. Lee was diagnosed with early-onset AD in 1996. Her *Just Love Me: My Life Turned Upside-down by Alzheimer's* (2003) recounts how she struggles with quiet heroism to maintain her life. Here is how she confronts an issue pertinent to step 5. Jeanne is very much a 'people person', who used to 'prefer groups of people, the more the merrier. Now I prefer not to have too many people around because of my difficulty with group conversation... Something that I...find disturbing...is that I have to frequently interrupt, because, if I don't, by the time they're finished with their story I've forgotten what I wanted to add' (p.32). Jeanne has learned to do this tactfully, but it's still hard for her to avoid uncomfortably feeling that she is rude.

As for myself, when I am in Jeanne's situation and am deciding whether to interrupt, I might infer from my interlocutors' tones of voice (to which AD has increased my sensitivity) that their contribution is winding down, and I can safely memorize my contribution while practically tuning them out. But I risk being mistaken and finding that I end up losing both the conversational thread and my potential contribution.

To further illustrate my belief that rehabilitation is possible, I will draw on Gottman and DeClaire's *The Relationship Cure* (2001). This book is full of examples where painful disconnection between persons is overcome through sensitive and clever conversational initiatives – difficult, of course, for us PWiDs whose minds go blank under stress. However, persons with mild dementia are notorious for learning the social skills to disguise their condition. And, having observed Yehuda Ben-Yishay's work (2000) at Rusk Institute with patients with brain injuries much more severe than mild AD, I believe this capacity for learning can be extended to compensate for deficits, not merely disguise them.

Here is an example of a situation that might be problematic for PWiDs. It shows a failed connection between a 'jester', one who specializes in conversational contributions that are entertaining, and a nest-builder, one who specializes in contributions fostering bonding and affiliation.

Nest-builder: I can't believe you told that joke in front of the board members. What if you offended somebody?
Jester: Oh, relax! People laughed didn't they? That's what matters.
(Exchange ends on an uncomfortable note.)
                                        (Gottman and DeClaire 2001, pp. 133–4)

Let's assume the nest-builder is a PWiD. (PWiDs often develop their nest-building skills and interests to compensate for the loss of their more aggressive competences.) What would it take for her not to be shoved aside by an obdurate TAB jester, but to stand up for her concern? (Another pertinence of this example is that PWiDs are newly being encouraged to participate on the boards of Alzheimer's Associations.) Gottman proposes the nest-builder rejoin with:

Of course they laughed. You've got such a wild sense of humor! but I guess it's just the way I'm wired – I'm always worried about whether something might hurt somebody's feelings. Do you think it would be all right if I checked in with a few key people to see if any apologies are needed?

Jester: Sure, if that will make you feel better, go ahead.

(Exchange ends on a peaceful note.)

(Gottman and DeClaire 2001, pp.133–4)

The nest-builder is (1) mirroring the jester's positive intent, then (2) remarking on the jester's corresponding enduring attribute. Then (3) the nest-builder, a little disarmingly, self-discloses about her own temperament, and (4) a bit tentatively proposes a typical nest-building action. (Note that, fortunately, none of this requires the nest-builder to remember any details of the joke or to make complex improvisations on the spot.) The social skill involved requires training, of course. The four steps can be practised separately and then combined. Step 2 is an important part of the Rusk program, and their impressive results suggest that the full package ought to be practicable.

Conclusion

Although it is not usual, there are sufficient instances of PWiDs making pleasant sustained social connections with TABs through mutual good will, understandings and adjustments to verify that 'Tedious no more!' is a realistic goal for us, just as it is for developmentally disabled persons. As I indicated above, by referring to the ghetto and the Holocaust, this project has overtones transcending the domain of comfortable sociability. The southern black struggle to sit at lunch-counters was more than a matter of nutrition. Whenever a person who is weak affirms his or her human dignity everyone else who is poor, weak or oppressed stands to benefit.

Notes

1   A general step by step approach to rehabilitation is presented in Friedell 2003.

2   See members.aol.com/morrisff/AlzAnon.html for an 'Alzheimer's Anonymous' program I sketched.

    Self-awareness: Brach (2003) *Radical Acceptance* is thoughtful and readable. It is written from a Buddhist perspective. See also Davis (2002) *The Divorce Remedy* and Gendlin (1982) *Focusing.* Self-reflection: I suggest Covey, Merrill and Merrill (1994). Self-determination: Setters (2002) *Trophy Wives* has an interesting treatment of this. (PWiDs aren't the only ones who need to struggle to avoid being 'surface'.) Judd (1999) is good on journaling in neuropsychological rehabilitation. Self-appreciation: I suggest Sinetar (1987). Schnarch (1997) *Passionate Marriage* is good on constructive self-expression in tense relationships (self-expression) and on the systole and diastole of challenge (the first 5 steps) and comfort (self-acceptance). Sex is Schnarch's topic, and here TABs are usually as awkward as PWiDs are in other areas.

References

Ben-Yishay, Y. (2000) 'Postacute neuropsychological rehabilitation.' In A.-L. Christensen and B.P. Uzzell (eds) *International Handbook of Neuropsychological Rehabilitation*. New York: Kluwer Academic/ Plenum Publishers.

Brach, T. (2003) *Radical Acceptance*. New York: Bantam.

Cohen, D. and Eisdorfer, C. (2001) *The Loss of Self: A Family Resource for the Care of Alzheimer's Disease and Related Disorders* (revised and updated edn). New York: Norton.

Covey, S., Merrill, A.R. and Merrill, R.R. (1994) *First Things First*. New York: Simon and Schuster.

Davis, M. (2002) *The Divorce Remedy*. New York: Simon and Schuster.

Friedell, M. (2000) 'Potential for Rehabilitation in Alzheimer's Disease' (available at members.aol.com/morrisff/Rehab.html) was presented as a poster at the World Alzheimer Congress in Washington, DC, 2000.

Friedell, M. (2003) 'Dementia Survival – A New Vision.' *Alzheimer's Care Quarterly* April/June, 79–84.

Gendlin, E. (1982) *Focusing*. New York: Bantam.

Gottman, J. and DeClaire, J. (2001) *The Relationship Cure*. New York: Three Rivers Press.

Henderson, C. (1998) *Partial View: An Alzheimer's Journal*. Dallas: Southern Methodist University Press.

Judd, T. (1999) *Neuropsychotherapy and Community Integration*. New York: Kluwer Academic/ Plenum Publishers.

Killick, J. and Allan, K. (2001) *Communication and the Care of People with Dementia*. Philladelphia: Open University Press.

Lee, J. (2003) *Just Love Me: My Life Turned Upside Down by Alzheimer's*. West Lafayette, IN: Purdue University Press.

Mitchell, G. and Jonas-Simpson, C. (2003) *Countering Stigma with Understanding: Listening to Persons Diagnosed with Dementia*. Unpublished manuscript.

Rauschi, T.M. (2001) *A View from Within: Living with Early Onset Alzheimer's*. Albany, NY: Northeastern New York Chapter Alzheimer's Disease and Related Disorders Association.

Schnarch, D. (1997) *Passionate Marriage*. New York: Henry Holt.

Setters, C. (2002) *Trophy Wives*. Xlibris Corporation, www.Xlibris.com.

Sinetar, M. (1987) *Do What You Love, The Money will Follow*. New York: Dell.

CHAPTER 8

Some Views of People with Dementia

The PROP Group

Since 2000 a small team of professionals in the Doncaster area has been working with younger people with dementia and their carers to ascertain the needs of this distinct client group and to ensure that as services develop locally these needs are acknowledged and taken into account.

Service users have established the PROP Group (people relying on people), which has its own committee meetings to discuss the running of services and other issues. They attend a variety of stakeholder events to gather views and feed into service planning.

(Minutes of meeting with Janet Woodhouse of Dementia Collaborative, 25 February 2003)

The views of people with dementia with varying degrees of impairment have been sought. The content of these stories reflect the nature of the group they belong to and to the importance placed upon user involvement. Interviews were conducted by Denise Chaston, a clinical nurse specialist, who founded the PROP Group along with a carer.

Interviews

MC is a 51-year-old man who recently moved back into the local area from a big city where he worked as a social worker.

I describe rehabilitation as being able to live in one's own home and to be helped to live life as normally as possible. It's also important to get help in coming to terms with your difficulties.

I have always felt that professionals should bother to provide rehabilitation for people with memory problems: it is worthwhile. During my working life I would do my best to provide this and attempted to delay institutionalization for as long as possible.

Community care is of paramount importance, community resources should be used to the full to maintain and encourage people with memory problems. It's about talking to people and helping them get on with their lives, not just about the physical care such as bathing and toileting. I feel that appropriate language must be used, we must be able to understand what is being said to us and people should take time with us.

When I was first diagnosed I had lots of input from different people in the professions, then I was left and this is why we moved back to the local area, to be nearer family and friends. I find it extremely difficult to come to terms with my difficulties because the shoe is on the other foot now. It can be very difficult to accept help when people are telling you what to do. I am now fortunate that the group that I go to involves both users and carers in the care that is planned and delivered. I am actually asked what I want and that feels good, I feel as though I am worth listening to again.

JD is a 59-year-old man who has been a very active member of a political party, a trade union rep and worked in management for the local authority.

Rehabilitation to me means that you need plenty of activity to keep your mind on the go. You must not sit and brood and that way you feel valued and included. You must have a purpose to get up and you don't want to vegetate. Rehabilitation helps you to keep positive and enjoy yourself. I'm told that my brain is deteriorating but I won't throw in the towel. Why shouldn't people with memory disorders get rehabilitation, other people do with other conditions such as stroke; they have active rehabilitation both physically and mentally so why not us – it's just the same? The group I'm involved with has helped. I have to look in my diary to see what events I've got coming up. I feel that since I've become active I feel that my brain has compensated to do some tasks that I used to forget such as leaving keys in doors. I know it might be wishful thinking but I think the activities help me so I join in with everything.

I had to finish work because of my diagnosis and then it was nothing, I don't want to go into an older persons centre, I saw what institutionalization did when I was working as I had to inspect older persons' facilities. It's so important to have someone to help, someone very pro-active and creative, someone who will give you that encouragement when you need it. Yes, I do think that rehabilitation for people with memory problems is worthwhile.

BP is a 62-year-old woman who previously worked in the printing trade.

BP: Rehabilitation – I am not really sure what that means.

Denise: Ok, I will try to explain what it means. When someone breaks their leg they get rehabilitation, usually from a physiotherapist, to get them going again. So it's about allowing a person to achieve their potential. Do you think that you have had any rehabilitation?

BP: I have always been a sociable person but when the diagnosis of dementia was made this affected my confidence and I felt that people saw me as a problem. I disappeared. I think I am lucky that I have been seen by a physiotherapist who has helped me to help with my walking, a social worker visited me to look at my benefits and I have you, who persuaded me to join in with the young onset group. We sat down to talk about what activities I enjoy doing and you arranged for a befriender to visit me. She helps to support me when I undertake the activities. Very soon I am moving to another area of the country and I want the same there as I have here.

MB is 64 years old and previously worked in a jewellers.

Denise: Do you enjoy coming to the group?

MB: Yes, I do.

Denise: Why is that?

MB: I like seeing people like me and I like to watch what is going on and join in.

Denise: People like you?

MB: Yes, people that have problems with their memory, I'm always forgetting, you know what I'm like.

Denise: So it's good to mix with other people with the same problems as you?

MB: Yes, I don't feel stupid if I make a mistake and sometimes I help other people. That makes me feel good.

Denise: What do you like doing best of all?

MB: What do I do, can you remind me?

Denise: You go out on trips. The last one was to Beamish Museum. You also go on holidays.

(At this point MB was shown photos of these events.)

MB: Oh, yes.

Denise: Do you enjoy these activities?

MB: Yes. The museum made me remember things and I enjoyed telling the children who came with us about how things used to be.

Denise: What would you do if you didn't come here?

MB: Sit at home or in the garden, not much. I am glad I come to the group, I am not on my own.

Denise: Is it worth people with memory problems taking part in activities?

MB: Yes, we are not finished with just yet!

CHAPTER 9

Our Views on Rehabilitation

Tom and Sheila Davis

Sheila

I am Sheila Davis and I am 79 – 80 in October. I developed dementia which seemed very slow in creeping on. Housework helps and keeps you busy and keeps the muscles moving. I have got friends who have helped a lot and still feel I can carry on with their help and laughter in between! I can't drive any more and I miss that but have a good husband who helps with the shopping, etc. I would like to be more independent but he is very helpful.

The family are very good but don't fuss – they are mostly away so that means I look forward to their visits. It is a very different attitude and outlook once your outlook changes and you accept dementia – a lot of it can be fun!!

Tom

Shattered! Absolutely shattered! That was my immediate emotional feeling when the consultant told us that my lovely wife (Sheila) was diagnosed as being in the early stages of dementia.

'To rehabilitate' – I looked this up in the dictionary and briefly it is 'to help someone who has been seriously ill to readapt to society,' i.e. to restore them to normality. How can you do this with dementia? I also looked up dementia: 'a state of serious mental deterioration'. So the two words are opposites, how can you revert to normal a condition that is on a never-ending downward curve? However, having got that off my chest, how were we going to deal with it?

Well – we sat down and we talked and cried and talked and cried, took a deep breath and decided that all the family and close friends were to be told and brought into the equation so that they would be forewarned if Sheila was ever in a confused state in their presence, and a very good decision it was. In hindsight (and what a right clever devil he is) Sheila's condition had been creeping up on us for a few years and I feel mortified now when I look back at the times when I have been irritated by some silly little lapse in her behaviour.

We have both always had a very good sense of humour and this above anything else has proved to be a boon. In our ordinary day-to-day life we really do laugh at some of Sheila's little mishaps and there are many in the course of a day.

On a practical level, I have made all electrical switches and appliances as safe as possible and I have had the cooker taken out because Sheila was burning her arms on the grill. We have replaced the cooker with an up-to-date microwave but this has its limitations in respect of producing a good nourishing meal. To offset this we now have lunch out three times a week to ensure a good balanced diet and have a light evening meal that can be prepared on the electric hob.

Sheila has as much independence as possible, e.g. I go to the supermarket with her and push the trolley but she makes all the decisions on what we purchase. Sheila is not comfortable about being out on her own and has from time to time forgotten her name, but she does have days out with friends and comes home recharged and full of chat. I ensure that I have time to myself to pursue my own hobbies and all in all we seem to have the balance about right.

Finally, the best therapy we have for Sheila is Charlie the dog. He is a miniature dachshund, absolutely devoted to Sheila, and vice versa, so she is never really alone, and when I am out he is her companion and friend.

We did for a brief period try medication but Sheila had very bad side effects and we decided not to go any further down that road. We will just let nature take its course and deal with whatever conditions arise in our own way.

PART THREE

Specific Professional Perspectives

CHAPTER 10

The Role of Physiotherapy in Dementia Rehabilitation

Larissa Kempenaar

Introduction

Physiotherapists have historically been involved in the rehabilitation process of people with a wide variety of conditions, including neurological, musculoskeletal and cardiovascular conditions. The main role of physiotherapy in health care has been described by the Chartered Society for Physiotherapy as 'concerned with human function and movement and maximizing potential' (Chartered Society of Physiotherapy 2002). Physiotherapists use physical approaches to restore 'physical, psychological and social well-being, taking account of variations in health status' (Chartered Society of Physiotherapy 2002). As part of a multidisciplinary team, the physiotherapist can therefore make a valuable contribution to the rehabilitation of people with dementia.

This chapter will first provide an overview of the conditions physiotherapists may assess and treat in a dementia rehabilitation setting. Then it will discuss the principles of physiotherapy in the rehabilitation of people with dementia.

What conditions can physiotherapists assess and treat?

The majority of people with dementia are elderly. The conditions a physiotherapist may come across in dementia rehabilitation can therefore be divided into two groups: those physical problems commonly experienced by elderly people and those specifically related to dementia.

Musculoskeletal problems

A physiotherapist may be involved in the rehabilitation of musculoskeletal problems, i.e. problems in the muscles and joints. This can be divided into two groups of problems: first, those problems commonly associated with ageing, for example limitations associated with osteoarthritis such as limited movements, swelling, pain and associated muscle weakness; and second, the impairments associated with trauma, such as fractures, sprains and injuries. These are more frequent in people with dementia than in elderly people generally (Shaw *et al.* 2003) as cognitive impairment has been associated with an increased number of falls and increased mortality when a hip fracture has been sustained (Koustavlis and Wolfson 2000).

Mobility

The term mobility refers here to a transfer of the body, e.g. from lying to sitting, from sitting to standing or walking and turning. Mobility problems in people with dementia can have a variety of causes. First, the aforementioned musculoskeletal problems, for example weakness in the thigh muscles, can affect a person's gait or the ability to rise from a chair. Second, dementia has been associated with numerous physical symptoms, including Parkinsonian features such as rigidity, balance problems, problems with initiation of movement, visuospatial impairment (i.e. judging depth, height and length of spaces using eyesight), shuffling gait, loss of arm swing etc. Physiotherapists are able to provide specific exercises for these kinds of problems or may be able to provide the person with a mobility aid, such as a walking stick, a zimmer frame or a rollator. When a physiotherapist assesses a person's mobility, they will assess in the process the appropriateness of footwear (for example slippers, uncomfortable or worn out footwear will inhibit gait), furniture (for example, is the chair or bed of the right height?) and clothing (for example, length of trouser leg may get in the way).

Third, mobility problems can be based on a variety of symptoms indirectly associated with dementia. For example, decreased mobility may be related to a lack of motivation to mobilize as the person may not perceive a need to go anywhere. The person may experience fear when mobilizing as they have difficulty judging depth and height, for example when descending stairs. Fear and/or a reluctance to mobilize may also be experienced when entering spaces which are poorly lit, such as toilets, rooms or corridors. Commonly these fears are based on a lack of sensory information, leaving the person with dementia confused about their ability to move around in the environment.

Pain

Although the treatment of pain in dementia care deserves more than a single paragraph, it is important to mention pain in the context of rehabilitation and physiotherapy. Pain affects cognition, motivation and will affect how the person with dementia responds to any rehabilitative intervention. Those people with dementia who experience verbal communication impairments may not be able to report pain as easily and are particularly at risk of receiving insufficient medication and treatment of pain. It is therefore essential to ensure that pain is assessed and treated appropriately prior and during interventions to allow rehabilitation (Horgas 2003). Pain is one of the physical impairments physiotherapists assess and treat on a daily basis. The involvement of a physiotherapist with a person who is suspected to suffer from pain may therefore be recommended as they may be able to provide a non-drug intervention for pain, for example by using TENS (Transcutaneous Electrical Nerve Stimulation), gentle exercise or massage.

Many of the conditions described are not specific to dementia and the interventions employed by physiotherapists will therefore be similar to those employed in elderly care. However, the principles and approach employed by the physiotherapist in dementia rehabilitation will be specific to the needs of the person with dementia.

Principles of physiotherapy in dementia rehabilitation

Communication

As verbal communication may be impaired in people with dementia, the physiotherapist has to adjust communication to suit their needs. This may mean simplifying language when providing instructions, by using shorter sentences or alternative wordings. Alternatively, it may mean using non-verbal communication. This includes the use of touch, sound and vision. Touch can be used to communicate many things in physiotherapy, always keeping in mind that the person should consent to it. Touch can be used for directional guidance during walking, by placing the hand on the shoulder or literally by taking someone 'by the hand'. Touch can be used to facilitate movement by, for example, providing gentle pressure on the hips when someone sits down on a chair or by putting a hand on the lower back when rising from the chair. If a person requires considerably more help with walking or transferring, firmer support may be needed from one or two people. When the person experiences a fear of walking, support can be provided by walking closely with and in contact with the person. Touch can be used as a means of making initial contact with a person.

Sounds can be used to provide additional stimulation to enhance normal movement or to provide a signal. For example, a common problem in people with dementia is a decrease of the sense of body rhythm. This means that walking, which normally occurs in a regular rhythmic pattern, may appear irregular and, if a person already experiences balance problems, may become hazardous. Some people's gait improves by providing an external rhythm, by, for example, stamping the feet audibly, by counting out loud or by playing music with a rhythm appropriate to the speed of the person's gait. Sometimes gait improves by suggesting to the person the use of an internal rhythm, by asking them to count or sing to themselves. Alternatively, sounds can be used to trigger an appropriate response to an instruction. For example, when a person with dementia may not understand your wish to get them to sit down, it may be useful to pat the chair to provide an auditory signal.

Visual stimuli can be used to demonstrate the instructions. For example, when the person with dementia is expected to sit down, the physiotherapist may sit down at the same time as asking them to sit. When carrying out exercises, it is often more effective to demonstrate the exercise than to simply give the instructions.

For those who have recently started working with people with dementia or would like to have more specific instructions on how to mobilize a person with dementia, I would recommend the book by Rosemary Oddy (Oddy 1998).

Lateral thinking

One of the potential obstructions to the effectiveness of physiotherapy instructions is the person's short-term memory problems. Where in mainstream physiotherapy patients are expected to remember exercises, advice and previous treatments, this may not be possible in dementia rehabilitation. Compliance with physiotherapy intervention is therefore usually expected to be poor and the effect of treatment diminished. Alternative means have to be sought to aid the person's memory to carry out the exercises and advice.

To achieve the treatment goals set out following the physiotherapy assessment, it is essential to search for interventions which are suited to the person with dementia and the physiotherapist. The first option is to provide the person with dementia with memory aids for exercises. This can be done by providing exercise and advice sheets and by discussing with the person how they might best remember to use them. For example even when an exercise sheet is provided, unless it is hung up in a particular place where the person can regularly view this, it is likely that the exercises will be forgotten. Carers may have a useful role to play, whether they are the home help, friends or the family. The carer can be invited to participate, assist or remind the person with dementia to carry out the exercises or advice provided by the physiotherapist.

The second option is to choose the intervention to match the level of understanding of the person with dementia. As many people with dementia have degrees of aphasia and agnosia, it may be difficult to give the person verbal or visual instructions you would give to a patient without cognitive impairment. For example, if the problem identified is related to the person's cardiovascular fitness, it may be that ordinarily the patient would spent some time in the gym, using cardiovascular equipment such as an exercise bike or a treadmill. Some people with dementia may enjoy using this kind of equipment, however, due to agnosia the purpose and use of the equipment may be confusing. It may therefore be more beneficial to take the person for a walk, while ensuring the principles of cardiovascular training are applied by walking for the right length of time at a speed that should get them slightly out of breath. If the aim of treatment is to reduce the risk of the person falling by improving the person's standing balance, this can be done by providing the person with dementia with explicit exercises asking them to consciously work on balance. Alternatively, activities can be carried out with the person which indirectly challenge balance, for example by playing games with balls or activities such as dancing. In summary, it is important to achieve the rehabilitation goal, but *how* you achieve these depends on the abilities of the person with dementia, their carer and the physiotherapist.

The key to finding the right intervention for the person is using a person-centred approach (Kitwood 1997). This means that the person with dementia is not only seen as the patient with physical and neurological deficits, but as a unique person. By considering all aspects of the person, such as their life history, social background, personal likes and dislikes, and by viewing the physiotherapy goals as only part of the person's rehabilitation programme, it is possible to find effective interventions which will aid the person in achieving their goals.

Motor learning

The reality of physiotherapy in dementia rehabilitation is often that treatment only occurs when the physiotherapist is present, reducing the effectiveness of the intervention. This problem is common to physiotherapy with cognitively intact patients and is commonplace in dementia rehabilitation, despite efforts to overcome these problems. The evidence for the effectiveness of physical rehabilitation is, however, inconclusive. Most studies investigating the effectiveness of physical rehabilitation exclude people with cognitive impairment (Gillespie *et al.* 2003). One of the few studies which looked specifically at the effectiveness of physical rehabilitation for people with cognitive impairment was carried out by Shaw *et al.* (2003) who investigated the effectiveness of a multidisciplinary intervention for people with dementia after they presented with a fall at an A&E department. The outcome measure was the number of people with dementia who fell in the year following the intervention. Although the number of falls after the intervention (652, n=130) was smaller for the subjects in the intervention group when compared to the subjects in the control group (728, n=144) it was non-significant. No other differences were found between groups. One of the main limitations of this study is that the results were not analysed for subgroups of types of dementia. Subjects with Alzheimer's disease (AD), multi-infarct dementia (MID) and Lewy body dementia (LBD) were treated as one group. This may have skewed results as the intervention would not have been able to improve the risk or number of falls occurring as a result of transient ischaemic attacks (TIAs) in MID or as a result of neuronal loss in the brainstem (substantia nigra and locus coeruleus) in LBD.

On the contrary Huusko *et al.* (2000) did find evidence to support the effectiveness of rehabilitation for people with dementia. They carried out a randomized controlled trial to evaluate the effectiveness of rehabilitation of elderly people with hip fractures. A sub-analysis was carried out of the subjects with dementia, by categorizing subjects in four categories of cognitive impairment based on Mini Mental State Scores. They compared length of stay after a hip fracture for subjects in the experimental group who received intensive multidisciplinary rehabilitation and a control group who received treatment as normal. There was no significant difference between subjects with severe dementia or subjects without cognitive impairment in the experimental or control group. There was a significant reduction in length of stay between subjects with mild and moderate suspected dementia in the intervention group when compared to the control group, indicating that intensive rehabilitation benefits both people with and without dementia. When comparing subjects within the intervention group they found that the same percentage of people without dementia as with dementia was able to return to independent living following the same length of stay in hospital. Although the sub-analysis resulted in smaller samples in each group, the results indicate that rehabilitation can be effective for people with dementia.

The main difference between these studies appears to be the choice of outcome measure. Whereas it may be difficult to influence the number of falls of the person with dementia, in particular when not looking at specific sub-types of dementia, it was possible to reduce the length of stay in hospital for people with mild/moderate dementia following a hip fracture. Physical rehabilitation in dementia care is based on the learning or relearning of motor skills. As short-term memory and information retention is impaired in dementia, it could be assumed that learning of any skill in dementia would be impaired. However, based on the results of the Huusko *et al.* (2000) study, people with dementia appear to have sufficient motor learning skills to have rehabilitation potential. This is supported by research investigating motor learning skills in people with dementia. For example, Willingham *et al.* (1997) found that for subjects with Alzheimer's disease, although slower and less accurate than non-cognitively impaired controls at motor learning tasks, their learning of these motor skills was equivalent to that of controls. This may explain why people with Alzheimer's disease can still benefit from physical rehabilitation.

Conclusion

Although rehabilitation is the core aim of physiotherapy many people do not view physiotherapy in dementia care as rehabilitative. This may be the case, as the same degree of recovery as physiotherapists potentially achieve in an out-patient department or a stroke unit may not be achieved. Although restoration to previous function may not be feasible, the aim of rehabilitation should be to reduce the impact of dementia on the person's functioning and maximize the person's potential (Plant 2002). Evidence to support the effectiveness of physical rehabilitation is inconclusive, however, there is evidence to suggest that people with Alzheimer's disease are still able to learn new motor skills. A balance in physiotherapy in dementia rehabilitation should therefore be sought between an optimism in achieving optimal physical functioning and the reality that dementia is a progressive disorder, which will in time affect the person's physical functioning.

References

Chartered Society of Physiotherapy (2002) *The Curriculum Framework for Qualifying Programmes in Physiotherapy.* London: CSP.

Gillespie, L.D., Gillespie, W.J., Robertson, M.C., Lamb, S.E., Cumming, R.G. and Rowe, B.H. (2003) 'Interventions for preventing falls in elderly people.' *Cochrane Musculoskeletal Injuries Group, Cochrane Database of Systematic Reviews* Vol 1.

Horgas, A.L. (2003) 'Pain management in elderly adults.' *Journal of Infusion Nursing 26*, 3, 161–165.

Huusko, T.M., Karppi, P., Avikainen, V., Kautiainen, H. and Sulkava, R. (2000) 'Rehabilitation after hip fracture in patients with dementia.' *British Medical Journal 321*, 1107–1111.

Kitwood, T. (1997) *Dementia Reconsidered: The Person Comes First.* Buckingham: Open University Press.

Koustavlis, A.T. and Wolfson, C. (2000) 'Elements of mobility as predictors of survival in elderly patients with dementia: Findings from the Canadian Study of Health and Aging.' *Chronic Diseases in Canada 21*, 3, 93–103.

Oddy, R. (1998) *Promoting Mobility for People with Dementia: A Problem-solving Approach.* London: Age Concern England.

Plant, R. (2002) 'Rehabilitation concepts.' In A. Squires and M. Hastings (eds) *Rehabilitation of the Older Person: A Handbook for the Interdisciplinary Team* (3rd edn). Cheltenham: Nelson Thornes Ltd.

Shaw, F.E., Bond, J., Richardson, D.A., Dawson, P., Steen, I.N., McKeith, I.G. and Kenny, R.A. (2003) 'Multifactorial intervention after a fall in older people with cognitive impairment and dementia presenting to the Accident and Emergency Department: A randomised controlled trial.' *British Medical Journal 326*, 73–79.

Willingham, D.B., Peterson, E.W., Manning, C. and Brashear, H.R. (1997) 'Patients with Alzheimer's disease who cannot perform some motor skills show normal learning of other motor skills.' *Neuropsychology 11*, 2, 261–271.

Further reading

Donaghy, M. and Durward, B. (2000) *National Service Framework Mental Health Evidence-Based Briefing Paper: A Report on the Clinical Effectiveness of Physiotherapy in Mental Health.* London: Chartered Society of Physiotherapy.

Pomeroy, V. (1995) 'Dementia.' In T. Everett, M. Dennis and E. Ricketts *Physiotherapy in Mental Health.* London: Butterworth and Heinemann.

CHAPTER 11

Dementia in Primary Care: Think Rehab

Ian Greaves

General practitioners who are interested in dementia are few and far between. The results of the Audit Commission's *Forget Me Not* report (2000) shows that over half of a demoralized general practitioner workforce admits that they do not know enough about dementia. Only 48 per cent of GPs surveyed felt that they had received sufficient training to help them diagnose and manage dementia and only 54 per cent recognized the importance of actively looking for the early signs of dementia. Indeed, some GPs hold negative attitudes to the reporting of early diagnosis partly due to the distress evoked in patients by giving this bad news. So the message that needs to go out to primary care is that these patients are interesting, challenging and fun to treat and that a proactive caring approach can greatly enhance their quality of life. Think of rehabilitation so that your patients can get the most out of their lives.

As a family doctor I would consider it part of my role to help a patient who has suffered an amputation deal with the loss of their limb and help them with rehabilitation. The disability and need is obvious and my role may vary from advocacy to emotional and physical support. It took me a while to realize that I could and should provide similar services for patients with dementia. The disability is not so obvious but the principles remain the same. The aim is to make the most of what they have got, acknowledge their disability and treat them with respect.

Dementia is a syndrome with many causes. To make it easy to understand, think of it as brain failure. It then becomes manageable and can be put into a medical storage box and thought of as we do, for example, for patients who have heart failure. The brain and the heart are essential organs and failure of function has some dramatic effects. Doctors often think that dementia is only a problem where the patient has memory lapses. However, dementia has three main expressions:

1.   Cognitive deficits. This starts as a reduction in short-term memory, euphemistically called 'senior moments'. Most people develop compensation mechanisms such as confabulation or social ritual or become grumpy. In fact it can be difficult to spot early changes – most of my friends say they would not know the difference if I became demented. There are also changes in the ability to perform and interact socially. Again early changes are difficult to spot and show as an inability to make skilled movements and difficulty in interpreting sensations correctly. The reduction in verbal reasoning and loss of language skills can result in social isolation.

2.   Non-cognitive features such as depression, hallucinations, delusions, misidentifications and behavioural disturbances that are typified by agitation, aggression, wandering and sexual disinhibition. Behavioural changes with wandering, aggression and inappropriate behaviour usually herald a stage where coping at home becomes impossible and the patient is shipped off to a nursing home.

3.   Further deterioration of brain function then impacts on acts of daily living and results in dependence on others to look after them to survive. The patient presents with difficulties in feeding, dressing, toileting and activities such as using money, shopping or making telephone calls.

So where do GPs find a role in the rehabilitation of patients with dementia? Well, first, spot it early and give social, physical and practical support. Overcome the fears – remember the amputee. It would be a poor GP who let a patient with a loss of limb feel there is no future.

Most GPs with an average list size of about 2000 will have about one or two patients a year with a new diagnosis of dementia and, with a prevalence rate of 3.6, this is by no means a common or pressing problem. Unfortunately there are a lot more cases that will be unknown to the health care services. As a rule of thumb the incidence of dementia doubles within each decade of life over 60. Only 1 per cent of 60–64 year olds are affected, whereas dementia can be diagnosed in approximately 30 per cent of all people aged 90. The increased longevity and baby boomer social demographics mean that dementia is going to become more of a problem in the future. Although the incidence is relatively low compared to, say, chest infections or cardiovascular disease, patients with dementia are an enormous drain on our resources and time. Several agencies are usually involved in the care programme and the care plans require good communication and multidisciplinary working practices. Good rehabilitation demands that care plans involve the GP and his team.

Rehabilitation starts with helping people come to terms with their loss and the care plans should start to address the fears and feelings of the patients, relatives and their carers. It is very important to diagnose and start rehabilitation early and this is certainly in the domain of the general practitioner.

Common presentations

The most common presentation is by concerned relatives or neighbours with the demand for urgent action by the GP because of their fears for the patient's safety. The phrase that brings a feeling of dread to most GPs is 'something must be done about Tom, doctor'. It is often very distressing for relatives to see the progressive changes in cognitive ability and social function of someone they love and admire. Late presentations by relatives who have come to the end of their tether means that there is a sense of urgency and you have to deal with their feelings of guilt, despair and fear as well as the needs of the patient with dementia. This presentation may not come directly to the GP but through other members of the primary health care team, such as health visitors or practice nurses. Wardens who look after people in sheltered accommodation may report changes in behaviour or deterioration in the ability of their charges to perform acts of daily living. Sometimes the patient may only be drawn to your attention with a request for your input from another agency such as social services or the voluntary agencies such as the Alzheimer's Society. This could be in the form of a request to complete the medical assessment form for care plans or residential home placement.

Another common presentation is the request to visit patients in residential homes when there has been a deterioration in their mental health. The staff report that they cannot cope with abnormal behaviour and want you to refer for a psychiatric assessment or prescribe some form of sedation.

One of the most difficult presentations is to deal with a telephone call from the police because one of your patients has been found wandering in the night. The relatives and police see this as urgent and it is often time consuming and difficult for the GP to impress this same view on the other agencies. It is in situations like this where we need to work together as a team to overcome everyone's frustrations and fears. Compare how long it takes to admit someone with chest pain against a patient with behavioural problems due to dementia.

The lucky patients may be detected early either in screening clinics such as the over 75 checks or by yourself as part of the routine consultations as the family doctor. GPs see a lot of older people regularly for other conditions.

Why do patients present late?

1. Fear – there is nothing more frightening at any stage of life than to think that you may lose your mind.

2. Nothing can be done –'there are no treatments that work. If you do not want to know the answer then don't ask the question.'

3. Social fragmentation – elderly people who only see their relatives on limited occasions may easily deteriorate and this is only picked up at Christmas or family functions.

4. Fear of nursing homes – 'if I go to the doctor they will say I have got to go into a nursing home – I would rather die.'

5. Stigma – 'I don't want the social round here. What will people say?'

6. Cost – 'I have worked all my life to save something for the kids – I am not losing it all now.'

7. Intergenerational tensions – 'it's not fair on my children, they have their own lives to run.'

8. Senior moments – 'everyone gets forgetful as you get older, you expect it, don't you?'

9. Stubbornness – 'you cannot make me. I was born here and I will die here.'

10. Belief that they are 'not too bad' – 'I am all right, I don't believe that I left the cooker on – I can't remember that.'

Think rehab in early dementia

Early detection can really help in the rehabilitation of people with dementia. Firstly there is a new range of drugs – acetylcholinesterase inhibitors. These increase the level of acetylcholine in the brain by blocking the enzyme that breaks this chemical down. The easy way to look at this is as a brain stimulant. However, we need a brain to stimulate. These drugs therefore seem to work better if we can get them in earlier. Unfortunately the average time between suspecting that the patient may have dementia and being properly diagnosed can be several years. It seems that this is like clot busting in heart attacks and the greatest benefit is giving it early. Early diagnosis is also helpful in planning services for individuals, including treatments for non-cognitive symptoms. These should include psychosocial approaches. Independence can be maintained by environmental manipulation. Social interaction can be improved with activity programmes and other interventions. Remember that as GPs we can cure few but care for everyone. So as family doctors we should guide and signpost carers and relatives to all the appropriate agencies. We should ensure that there is a menu of services and therapies that are available to the family. Care plans change with disease progression and should be regularly reviewed.

How can we detect dementia early?

This is difficult but not impossible. Firstly we need to get the message out that early presentation helps. The target population are the elderly groups. In our area we go and talk to old people's clubs and social functions. If GPs cannot afford the time then there are plenty of volunteers in the Alzheimer's Society. The message needs to be upbeat and exciting to combat the negative image that is out there at present.

We can also use our position as family doctors. Elderly people are seen much more often than other patients and if GPs don't see them there are others in the primary health care team who do. The over 75s get seen by someone at least once a year. It's a case of having the suspicion and knowing the patients well. What you are looking for is change. Remember some of the brighter people can cover a considerable change in their cognitive powers whilst others may have less of a change, but the fall off takes them below the coping level and it is more noticeable. This is an excellent excuse for sitting down and having that cup of tea or sherry with the retired barrister – how else can you spend long enough to establish a rapport?

Spot the usual suspects

We are screening everyone now for cardiovascular disease. This seems to keep the government happy and pay the mortgage. Those at a high risk of arteriosclerosis are also at a high risk of vascular dementia. These high-risk patients regularly get examined and have bloods taken for baseline renal and lipids levels. They may even undergo an ECG, as it is easy then to spot the difference when they have an acute event. So why not add in a cognitive test? A fellow GP from Newbury, Patrick Brooke, promoted the simplest form of assessment called the 6 item cognitive impairment test (6 CIT) available at stjohnssurgery.co.uk/dementia. If we add this to the cardiovascular assessment we can use it to spot change. Remember that vascular dementia has a pattern of sudden declines and plateaus whereas Alzheimer's is gradual and progressive.

The Royal College of General Practitioners (2002) strongly recommend that GPs should identify dementia in older patients. In general they recommend that cognitive function be assessed in a systematic way. They recommend the following, but with a warning of cultural specificity:

1.   Ask the patient the time to the nearest hour. (Orientation)

2.   Give the patient an address to recall at the end of the test. The patient should repeat the address to ensure that it has been heard correctly. (Recall)

3.   Ask the patient to count backwards from 20 to 1. (Attention)

4.   Ask the patient to draw the face of a clock with the fingers pointing to ten to eleven.

5.   If the patient fails any of these go on to a full assessment.

Think rehab – secondary care or shared care

At present most of the people who have been diagnosed with dementia are referred to secondary care and in the majority of cases the service they get is excellent. The secondary care services, like us in primary care, are stretched to breaking point. It is unfortunate that over a third of the GPs in the *Forget Me Not* report felt that they did not have ready access to specialist advice. Specialist teams for older people with mental health problems were fully available in less than half of all areas and partly available in a further third. Most did not have a full complement of recommended core team members. The National Institute for Clinical Excellence put a further burden on these services by approving cholinesterase inhibitors for initiation only by specialists in mild to moderate Alzheimer's disease.

The common sense approach to all this would seem to be to help each other. The carve out model where a consultant assumes the care of a patient until they eventually die cannot be sustainable. Nor does the prevalence of the disease justify the transfer of memory clinics into primary care. Domiciliary visits increase costs and whilst giving the consultant first hand experience of the social arrangements of the patient may actually serve to lengthen waiting times. So the future of dementia care may be to come together to produce clearly defined pathways of care. This will serve to break down the tribal barriers of service provision, improve consistency and rapidity of diagnosis and set out best practice for management. This does not necessarily mean doing anything different – just smarter.

In our practice the adult psychiatrists run the out patient clinics at our surgery. This has reduced stigma and brought the services closer to the patient. The failures to attend have reduced from 30 per cent to 1 per cent. We GPs have gained confidence in the diagnosis and treatment of a lot of the common psychiatric problems and it is amazing how much is diffused subconsciously into a doctor's brain over a cup of coffee with a consultant colleague. Similarly the background information we have is vital and much better given verbally than in a three-page letter of referral. It is easy for us to help to prepare the patient for a consultant opinion, both in the physical work-up with the blood tests and other things that need to be done, and using our position as the trusted family doctor to help them understand the process and guide them through the multidisciplinary assessments that lie in front of them. We share resources – our practice nurses, community nurses, health visitors and their CPNs (community psychiatric nurses), EMI (elderly mentally ill) beds, respite services, day hospitals and other therapeutic options.

Surely this is the way forward for the elderly mentally ill? I am sure we should use joined up thinking to agree mutual pathways of care, with GPs doing the things we are good at, and get the best out of our consultant colleagues. It does not have to be as formal as outreach clinics. Perhaps we can agree to look at particular groups to get earlier identification of patients with suspected dementia and improve the quality of the referral with all the basic investigations done. We can monitor consultant initiated therapies and enact treatment plans. We do that for the diabetics and those patients who have cardiovascular disease. In turn the consultants would see our new referrals more quickly and bail us out if we phone them in a panic. This is not rocket science. Perhaps some of the CPNs could regularly visit the nursing homes and help us improve the lot of those patients with end stage dementia where the condition is much too severe for them to remain at home.

The social worker that visited our practice as part of a pilot for the scheme outlined above was bribed by coffee and compliments to stay on for a few days every week. She now has direct referrals and can sort out problems in days before they become chronic and enduring. Her case management has improved to deal with most problems within two or three days rather than six to nine months. In exchange we give her nursing and medical input and, more important, have began to understand her role and work with her as an integrated team.

The Department of Health is not going to commit a lot more funding to implement the National Service Framework (NSF) for older people. So it is up to us to do the best we can. Examples of best practice abound and the future of old age psychiatry lies in greater integration with primary care and social services.

Think rehab for the relatives and carers

The family and carers require special attention from the GP and good communication to enlighten and inform them about the disease and its effects on everyday life and social relations. Advice, signposting and advocacy regarding sources of care, service utilization, financial benefits and legal issues, including that of mental capacity, is required to guide them through the maze of service provision. Intergenerational tensions can become an obstacle to effective care plans unless handled with delicacy and sensitivity. Early planning to offer carer relief for family holidays and functions, combined with monitoring the impact of the burden of care, can help prevent carer fatigue. Respite care, day hospitals, befriending and sometimes a shoulder to cry on all have benefit. The voluntary bodies do remarkable work and a close working relationship with the Alzheimer's Society and other bodies can be enormously beneficial to the practice. There is a wealth of information available both in an electronic form and as newsletters and pamphlets. Guidelines published by European working groups and American societies may assist practical management.

Patient-centred rehab

Perhaps the best way to illustrate patient-centred rehab is to share with you a personal experience. My family hired the local village hall for a party for my mother's 90th birthday. She had about 50 friends who had survived to the fourth stage of life. As a special treat we engaged the services of the George Formby Society to come to entertain these old folks with some singing. It took an immense effort to get these people out of their homes and into the hall and they all sat around with vacant stares, occasionally speaking to one of the family as we dished out tea and cakes. Then the man from the society started. The atmosphere was transformed as tunes of yesteryear rang out. Feet were tapping and everyone who half an hour before looked disinterested joined in with the familiar lyrics. They were laughing and giggling at the saucy bits and the place and people were alive. They knew all the words and some even started to give me far too much information about the goings on at the local RAF camp during the war. The lesson here was obvious. Just as we need to teach the man with one leg to hop, we also need to engage the working portions of the brain in those with dementia. We should engage them in music, art and reminiscence therapies or whatever else we can do to let people communicate on their terms and conditions, not ours. Rehabilitation can be fun if you can get people to smile and enjoy themselves.

References

Audit Commission (2000) *Forget Me Not*. London: Audit Commission.

Royal College of General Practitioners (2002) *An Evidence-based Approach to Assessing Older People in Primary Care through the STEP Panel*. Occasional Paper 82, Royal College of General Practitioners..

CHAPTER 12

Rehabilitation after Acute Physical Illness

Peter Murdoch

Rehabilitation is concerned with enabling those with any short or longer-term disability to obtain the maximum degree of psychological and physical independence possible. The process should help people to 'be all they can be' and to enjoy life to the full. Physical rehabilitation following acute illness or other admission to acute hospital facilities is an especial challenge for people with dementia. This paper examines the reasons, challenges some of the prejudices and suggests positive measures to improve outcomes.

Low expectations

Andrews (1985) noted that rehabilitation is often complicated by low expectations (by staff rather than patients). In the 1980s and early 1990s, there was increasing evidence to support such staff pessimism. Lichtenberg *et al.* (1994) and Heinemann *et al.* (1994) were among those who found a clear association between cognitive impairment and poor functional outcome. People with dementia have increased risk of complications and a poor outcome from any co-existent physical problems or acute illness when compared to those without. For example, a person with dementia is three times as likely to have a fall and to sustain a fracture after any fall (Morris *et al.* 1987). If they do fracture a hip, on average they may stay for three times as long in hospital and are three times more likely not to be able to return home. Landi *et al.* (2002) found that cognitive impairment was the only significant negative predicting factor after intensive rehabilitation. Sauvaget *et al.* (2002) also confirmed that dementia was a strong predictor of functional disability. People with dementia who have had an amputation for vascular disease are significantly less likely to have a prosthesis successfully fitted (Fletcher *et al.* 2001). Seidel *et al.* (1994) confirmed that a person with dementia was significantly less likely to maintain urinary and faecal continence when compared with someone without cognitive impairment.

More positive experience

However, Hedman and Grafström (2001) explained that because of difficulties in assessing competence people with dementia are often erroneously judged as incapable of managing rehabilitation. Goldstein *et al.* (1997) reported positive outcomes of people with cognitive impairment who have had a hip fracture. Compared with their admission status, selected cognitively impaired hip fracture patients made significant overall motor improvements as well as specific functional gains in self-care, continence and mobility, although rehabilitation stays were longer. Gains, apart from mobility, were comparable to those without dementia. Cognitively impaired patients with mixed physical problems can also make significant gains in a geriatric rehabilitation unit. In stroke patients, dementia appears to account for only 12 per cent of variance in functional outcome (Hajek, Gagnon and Ruderman 1997). Ruchinskas, Singer and Repetz (2000) found that, in a study of urban geriatric rehabilitation patients with medical, neurological and orthopaedic diagnoses, although cognitive status has some effect on oral rehabilitative course and functional outcome, it does not predict walking or stair climbing ability. People with dementia do appear to benefit from rehabilitation after acute illness, although it may take longer.

Unnecessary or avoidable disability

The traditional negative attitude to rehabilitation of physical disability in people with dementia can become a self-fulfilling prophecy. Mary Marshall (1996) has written of the 'unnecessary disability' often engendered by acute hospital admissions. Possible contributory factors are:

- lack of awareness of cognitive impairment and special needs of those with it
- poor communication
- lack of training which may lead to inappropriate prescribing
- unnecessary investigation where results do not change management
- inadequate assessment due to under investigation
- a disabling and confusing environment
- undernutrition
- a bewildering process of care including multiple ward moves.

A Redesign Project at a District General Hospital in Scotland involved stakeholders, including patients, carers and health and social work professionals, within acute and community settings, in developing an integrated care pathway for people with dementia with acute physical needs (Forth Valley Redesign Project 2002). This proposed changes to previous practice in the community as well as within acute settings.

Community measures

A positive approach must start prior to any admission. There is a clear need for increased awareness and recognition of cognitive impairment in the community with attention to physical as well as psychosocial needs with appropriate intervention in the community. People with dementia should be included in health promotion programmes, including lifestyle advice and accident prevention. Regular physical activity helps to maintain mobility, general fitness and independence. If people with dementia require to be sent to acute hospital, whether as an inpatient or outpatient, essential information must be shared with hospital colleagues. Referrals should indicate if people do have some degree of underlying cognitive impairment. This is as crucial as noting any major relevant past medical history, current medication or history of serious drug allergy. It facilitates setting of realistic goals, better discharge planning, highlights the need for extra attention to communication with patients and carers, and expedites placement in the most positive environment for further therapeutic input within hospital.

When people with significant cognitive impairment live alone at home and also have physical problems, ensuring adequate information in the event of crisis is particularly valuable. One way of ensuring this is to keep basic information with name of care or next of kin in a readily accessible place, for example, in a tube in the fridge, so this can be accessed by emergency services and shared with acute colleagues if necessary. It is hoped that progress with single shared assessments between health and social work personnel of older people and those with dementia, as well as improvements in information systems, will result in better sharing of information essential to care and rehabilitation of such people.

Initial screening

Staff in Accident and Emergency departments as well as assessment units should screen all new attendees and admissions for cognitive or functional impairment (Clinical Standards Board for Scotland 2002). This enables identification of those at special risk and in special need of comprehensive social and functional assessment, especially regarding fall prevention (Tinetti and Speechley 1989). The balance of frail patients with dementia can be improved by appropriate training programmes (Toulotte *et al.* 2003). People with advanced dementia are also at substantial risk for undetected or undertreated pain (Morrison and Siu 2000).

Partnership

Successful rehabilitation is dependent on an effective partnership between the individual patient and their carers and the relevant health and social work professionals. It is no less important for those with dementia that there is common understanding of home circumstances; usual functional, cognitive, social and psychological attainment; and realistic shared goals of treatment and rehabilitation. Family members can often provide crucial background information to assist staff make a correct diagnosis and plan eventual successful discharge. The needs of carers, especially family members sharing the same residence, should also be addressed. Choice, dignity and autonomy should be respected and maximized in those with cognitive impairment even in hospital, but this requires good communication.

Communication

Communication between various members of the multidisciplinary team providing care and rehabilitation in hospital is vital. Extra time and attention is required to ensure clear communication with the person with dementia and their carers. Porters and domestic staff appreciate advice as much as others, for example X-ray department staff or phlebotomists, who may schedule more time to allow adequate reassurance and unhurried explanation of potentially frightening interventions.

Staff training and education

Lack of training and education about dementia may result in professional staff being unsure, hesitant or afraid and either prescribing inappropriately or taking too negative an approach. Provision of simple information on dementia and basic education about the special needs of people with the condition is very worthwhile and appreciated by all disciplines working in an acute hospital (Archibald 2002). Greater understanding of the causes of agitation or aggression encourages use of simple non-drug measures to relieve anxiety and calm patients. Awareness of the high incidence of delirium and depression in such circumstances, together with the confidence to recognize and treat these appropriately can greatly improve outcomes of acute treatment and rehabilitation. Appreciation of the increasing range of potential support at home and the importance of a familiar environment can enable hospital-based staff to discuss balance of risk and look into increased support at home, if this is a feasible option.

Whilst all staff working with adults in an acute setting require basic appreciation and understanding of dementia, especial interest and expertise should be encouraged within rehabilitation settings amongst medical, nursing and allied health professionals. Physical performance measures of strength and function can be reliably and usefully assessed in older people with dementia (Thomas 2002). Specialist techniques have for instance been developed within physiotherapy to maximise the benefits of such remedial therapy. Oddy (1998) described a problem-solving approach to promote mobility for people with dementia. Making communication easier, especially using non-verbal techniques such as touch and gesture; managing fear; improving the environment and advising family and other carers appear to improve outcomes.

An enabling environment

Simple measures can enable the environment to be less disturbing, improved lighting and clear signage to toilets, for example. Large clocks and reminders about the time and place are reassuring. It is important also to recognize other sensory impairments such as poor vision and hearing and seek to minimize these.

Fluids and nutrition

People with dementia are often unable to maintain adequate fluid and dietary intake to speed recovery and increased awareness is required from nurses, dieticians and domestic staff to maximize this. Hospital catering increasingly involves individually packaged cartons or portions, and those most at risk may leave meals untouched because of inability to unwrap them. Those with decreased thirst and at greatest risk of fluid depletion require ready access to appropriate drinks and careful supervision and monitoring. Staff in Falkirk Royal Infirmary developed a simple traffic lights approach to indicate those needing especial supervision or support. Those with cognitive impairment and acute illness, e.g. infection or stroke, are especially likely to have problems with safe swallowing and again need necessary specialist assessment and support.

A smoother pathway – improved processes

Finally, the process of care needs to be co-ordinated and smooth to ensure attention to careful discharge planning and a positive rehabilitative focus from the moment that a person with dementia enters hospital. Dr J. George in Carlisle has concentrated inpatient facilities for people with dementia with physical illness within a specific unit within an acute hospital to make best use of available skills and provide a positive approach to acute care and rehabilitation (personal communication). Elsewhere interest and limited expertise about dementia may be concentrated in a few key areas, such as geriatric rehabilitation, stroke or orthopaedic rehabilitation. Slaets *et al.* (1997) have shown the benefit of psychogeriatric liaison intervention in elderly medical in-patients and such specialist expertise appears to reduce institutionalization. The best local model may depend on local availability of rehabilitation facilities and clinical champions. Stakeholders should be encouraged to look at improving the pathway of care for all people with dementia and physical problems, be they medical, surgical or orthopaedic, in their local healthcare system.

Intermediate care

Webber (2003) was concerned that people with dementia were often excluded from rehabilitation in intermediate care facilities for rehabilitation and prevention of dependence on institutional care. However, they found that such patients may participate effectively in and benefit from such rehabilitation. It is as important that people with cognitive impairment are not excluded from such facilities as people with dementia having timely access to acute hospital facilities if required. In general, however, rehabilitation from relatively minor acute illness may be more effective if necessary support can be provided at home.

Conclusion

A great deal can and must be done to improve the acute care and rehabilitation of people with dementia, so that they can maximize their function, independence and general well-being after any physical illness. People with dementia have special needs, which if recognized and understood, can be addressed successfully with clear benefit to themselves, their carers and health and social care systems. Positive partnerships, focused on meeting such needs, enable those with both dementia and physical disability to be included in, rather than excluded from, effective programmes of rehabilitation.

References

Archibald, C. (2002) *People with Dementia in Acute Hospital Settings.* Stirling Dementia Services Development Centre.

Andrews, K. (1985) 'Rehabilitation of conditions associated with old age.' *International Rehabilitation Medicine 7*, 3, 125–129.

Clinical Standards Board for Scotland (2002) *Standards for Older People in Acute Care.* Edinburgh: CSBS.

Fletcher, D.D., Andrews, K.L., Butter, M.A., Jacobsen, S.J., Rowland, C.M. and Hallett, J.W. Jr. (2001) 'Rehabilitation of the geriatric vascular amputee patient.' *Archives of Physical Medical and Rehabilitation 882*, 6, 776–779.

Forth Valley Redesign Project (2002) *Development of Care Pathways for People with Dementia who have Intercurrent Physical Illness.* Final report. Falkirk: NHS Forth Valley.

Goldstein, F.C. Stasser, D.C., Woodard, J.L. and Roberts, V.J. (1997) 'Functional outcome of cognitively impaired hip fracture patients on a geriatric rehabilitation unit.' *Journal of the American Geriatrics Society 45*, 11, 1406–1407.

Hajek, V.E., Gagnon, S. and Ruderman, J.E. (1997) 'Cognitive and functional assessments of stroke patients: An analysis of their relation.' *Archives of Physical Rehabilitation 78*, 12, 1331–1337.

Heinemann, A.W., Linacre, J.M., Wright, B.D., Hamilton, B.B. and Granger, C. (1994) 'Prediction of rehabilitation outcomes with disability measures.' *Archives of Physical Medicine and Rehabilitation 75*, 133–143.

Landi, F., Bernabei, R. Russo, A., Zuccalà, G., Onder, G., Carosella, L., Cesari, M. and Cocchi, A. (2002) 'Predictors of rehabilitation outcomes in frail patients treated in a geriatric hospital.' *Journal of the American Geriatrics Society 50*, 4, 679–684.

Lichtenberg, P.A., Christensen, B., Metler, L., Nanna, M., Joans, G., Reyes, J. and Blumenthal, F. (1994) 'A preliminary investigation of the role of cognition and depression in predicting functional recovery in geriatric rehabilitation patients.' *Advances in Medical Psychotherapy 7*, 109–124.

Marshall, M. (1996) *'I Can't Place this Place at All.'* Birmingham: Venture Press.

Morris, J.C., Rubin, E.H., Morris, E.J. and Mandel, S.A. (1987) 'Senile dementia of the Alzheimer type: An important risk factor for serious falls.' *Journal of Gerontology 42*, 4, 412–417.

Morrison, R.S. and Siu, A.L. (2000) 'A comparison of pain and its treatment in advanced dementia and cognitively intact patients with a hip fracture.' *Journal of Pain Symptom Management 19*, 4, 240–248.

Oddy, R. (1998) *Promoting Mobility for People with Dementia: A Problem Solving Approach.* London: Age Concern England.

Ruchinskas, R.A., Singer, H.K. and Repetz, N.K. (2000) 'Cognition and ambulation in geriatric rehabilitation.' *Archives of Physical Medicine and Rehabilitation 81*, 1224–1228.

Rydholm-Hedman, A.M. and Grafström, M. (2001) 'Conditions for rehabilitation of older patients with dementia.' *Scandinavian Journal of Caring Sciences 15*, 2, 151–158.

Sauvaget, C., Yamada, M., Fujiwara, S., Sasaki, H. and Mimori, Y. (2002) 'Dementia as a predictor of functional disability: a four year follow-up study.' (Review) *Gerontology 48*, 4, 226–233.

Seidel, G.K., Millis, S.R., Lichtenberg, P.A. and Dijkers, M. (1994) 'Predicting bowel and bladder continence from cognitive status in geriatric rehabilitation patients.' *Archives of Physical Medicine and Rehabilitation 75*, 5, 590–593.

Slaets, J.P., Kauffmann, R.H., Duivenvoorden, H.J., Pelemans, W. and Schudel, W.J. (1997) 'A randomised trial of geriatric liaison intervention in elderly medical inpatients.' *Psychosomatic Medicine 59*, 6, 585–591.

Tinetti, M.E. and Speechley, M. (1989) 'Prevention of falls among the elderly.' *New England Journal of Medicine 320*, 1055–1059.

Thomas, V.S. (2002) 'Preliminary study on the reliability of physical performance measures in old care center clients with dementia.' www.Dementia.com

Toulotte, C., Fabre, C., Dangremont, B., Lensel, G. and Thevenon, A. (2003) 'Effects of physical training on physical capacity of frail demented patients with a history of falling.' *Age and Ageing 32*, 1, 67–73.

Webber, A. (2003) 'Rehabilitation of depressed and demented patients in intermediate care facilities.' Personal communication to BGS Spring Meeting.

CHAPTER 13

The Role of Occupational Therapy

Christine Davidson and Rona Bissell

As she was leaving the occupational therapy activity session at the day hospital Agnes said, 'I don't know what I did, but boy did I enjoy it'. It was music to our ears! That she is unable to recall the exact nature of the activity that occupied her for 45 minutes we believe to be inconsequential in this instance. What was important was that 'but boy did I enjoy it'.

Her statement is an expression of well-being, and the emotional response behind the statement includes those things associated with the concept of well-being. We consider these to be among the most valuable outcomes when working with people who have dementia. In terms of rehabilitative work with anybody, regardless of their abilities, what they are able to bring to and take from the therapy session, emotionally and psychologically, is one of the foundations on which we build.

Many people view those with the combined stigma of old age and mental illness as being of no further use to society and therefore unsuitable for rehabilitation. That they may have contributed to that society for many years is of no consequence. However, rehabilitation and therapy with this group of people can have a number of positive effects, not least increased well-being, personhood and decreased assistance required in activities of daily living, e.g. washing, dressing, cooking, watching TV, playing cards and so on.

Realigning perceptions of dementia

Dementia is often regarded as a degenerative illness leading to inevitable, irreversible deterioration. If a slight shift in emphasis is made to instead regard people with dementia as being people with a disability, then the concept of these people having ability is a simpler and logical step to make. The need to structure therapy and re-empower individuals to enhance personhood and to allow for 'rementing' (improvement that can take place when care is optimal) is formidable. And yet it remains an underrecognized area of expertise in occupational therapy.

Tom Kitwood (1997) when addressing notions of personhood and the social psychology of dementia, proposed that the individual was central; that their needs, abilities, goals and values should form the basis of any intervention. This concept of wholeness and individuality is one that is at the core of occupational therapy. This can be explained further by Elizabeth Yerxa, an American occupational therapist who is quoted as suggesting in 1967 that a person be seen 'not as an object or thing to be manipulated, controlled or made to conform but as a unique individual whose very humanness entitles him to choices determining his own destiny'. This is a sound basis for all therapeutic intervention. In order for a person to be engaged in a therapy and to experience gains through the therapeutic relationship it is imperative to have expectations of that individual, instances of this being that they have a free will, that they are able to communicate, respond, form opinions and change. Occupational therapists work alongside people to assist in finding the most appropriate and effective channels to achieve this self-determination, regardless of the level of disability.

Why occupational therapy?

The main thrust of occupational therapy is the philosophy of encompassing wholeness and individuality. Embedded in this philosophy are all the tenets that will provide necessary therapies to assist seamlessly in the assessment and necessary interventions of individuals. The use of graded activity by occupational therapists in the rehabilitation of individuals in health areas such as orthopaedics and stroke is well recognized and established. Quite simply these skills have been neither regularly applied nor fully exploited in relation to people disabled by dementia.

Stephen Wey (2000) looked at the concept of 'care of people with dementia' and suggested a change of focus toward 'therapy' and 'treating' the person who also happens to have dementia. His paper builds on the work of Vygotsky, a psychologist. It aligns his theories with the process of occupational therapy intervention with people who have dementia. In brief, this approach involves the theory of scaffolding. That is the sharing, validating, supporting and nurturing of individuals during their carrying out of any activity. This 'shoring up' can result in the emergence of self-determination, a sense of agency and increased occupational performance. Occupational therapy of this nature can incorporate a vast variety of interventions designed to both enhance personhood and to facilitate rementing.

Occupational therapy intervention uses activity and occupation in order to engage with people. Pierce (2001) describes these different concepts in the following terms:

> Activity is a one-dimensional concept, e.g. walking the dog, whereas occupation is all encompassing. It includes the emotions of carrying out the activity – breathing the fresh air, the smells, sights and sounds, where you're walking, with whom, the enjoyment (or otherwise), throwing toys for the dogs to retrieve.

The aim of our occupational therapy programmes is to enable the participants to be involved in occupation rather than activity: 'occupation is that which we possess and which possesses us' (Perrin and May 2000).

As occupational therapists we believe that occupation is essential for health and well-being. People with dementia are less able to seek out activity and fulfil their own occupational requirements. This can affect their ability to function as an individual within the context of their own home or as a member of a social group, e.g. a church. The progression from this may lead to hospitalization and/or relocation into the 'care' system. Further decline in occupational ability tends to follow this progression unless appropriate professional interventions are made.

Assessment

An occupational therapist can assess the individual, then analyse and examine the precise components of the activity that are becoming problematic. A programme of intervention can then be developed which is specific to the person and the task and is aimed at increasing the person's ability to take part in the task successfully. Occupational therapy uses several models and procedures to inform assessment, treatment planning and goal setting. One such model is the cognitive disability model. This model allows the therapist to assess the specific level at which the individual is functioning. Once this is known, a suitable treatment programme aimed at maintaining current functioning, probing for a higher level of functioning and maintaining/improving well-being can be devised.

In our experience one of the most effective occupational therapy assessments for this area of practice is observation, which may be perceived as less threatening than pencil and paper tests. Watching how someone carries out tasks and the skills and techniques they use to facilitate success is a good starting point for initiating therapy. People develop their own problem-solving strategies over time. We can use these as 'scaffolding' in order to assist people regain, improve and maintain skills.

There are occasions when an individual will be unsuccessful in carrying out a prescribed assessment or activity, no matter how much intervention and support is provided. At these times, if the individual displays distress at their perceived failure, an alternative activity can be explored. Alternatively the therapist can adapt the current activity to ensure some success is experienced. For example if someone is unable to complete the Allen's Cognitive Level Test (ACLT) (see Allen, Earhart and Blue 1992) leather lacing, this can be adapted into a sensory task – 'smell the leather; feel the rough and smooth surfaces'. We can still elicit valuable information, whilst protecting well-being by incorporating a 'feel good factor' regardless of the final product.

Intervention

Occupational therapists often cite maximizing independence as the principal aim for intervention. However, for people who are disabled by dementia, striving to achieve higher functioning tasks and well-being may not go hand in hand. For example, making a cup of tea: if the individual or their carer is concerned about injury and/or success and this is demonstrated through anxiety or other signs of ill-being in the person with dementia, then the question of continuing the activity and reinforcing the feelings of ill-being must be raised. We would need to examine alternative routes to involve the person in the task. Perhaps the carer does the main part of the activity, but gains assistance from the person to lay the table, find items and finish the activity, by pouring in the milk or offering biscuits. Interventions are carefully considered with the needs and wishes of the individual considered first and foremost.

Joan and George live in a rural community. Joan has severe dementia. The consultant psychiatrist expressed surprise at Joan's continued ability to function in her own home, albeit in a chaotic manner. George is struggling to cope and is frequently both frustrated and angry, failing to understand why she is unable to do things. Both reluctantly agree to an assessment by the occupational therapist, which revealed that Joan was desperate to maintain her position within the household and to continue to care for her husband as best she could. Within her home, Joan displayed difficulties due to perceptual problems, anxiety, reduced concentration and difficulties in problem-solving. She needed some levels of outside assistance with personal care, domestic assistance and day care. In order to maintain the family unit and to enhance Joan's well-being it was negotiated that Joan should have help in making meals for her husband three times a week. This support was designed to assist Joan in implementing the coping strategies developed by Joan, George and the occupational therapist.

We have used horticulture to elicit improvement of skills and well-being in people. For example, in the day hospital, individuals can successfully plant out a garden box in the spring. As time moves on towards summer plants are watered and nurtured. There are opportunities for reminiscence and reality orientation and there is reinforcement of the achievement in taking part in the task. There is discussion with and feedback from peers resulting in increased self-esteem and motivation.

Frequently in residential environments, the following decreasing spiral can occur, resulting in individuals becoming institutionalized. An individual is perceived to struggle with a task, or is slow to complete it, staff then take over and do the task, 'to help the person'. The person being helped no longer has the opportunity to practise the task, resulting in falling skill levels. This 'helping' is easily extended to cover all aspects of daily living, including the making of simple decisions by the helper on behalf of the person – brown bread or white? The 'doing for' and 'deciding for' become a formidable synergy against the person – not allowed to decide, can't do it anyway, time to switch off!

In order to address these possible issues a teatime group was established on the continuing care ward. The setting was relaxed with plenty of time and lots of choice in a quiet, homely environment. David was one of our four regulars. He had difficulty communicating, and very rarely did so verbally. He also showed little awareness of others. At one group, several weeks into the intervention he turned to his neighbour and offered half a scone 'this is for you, Tom'. This was appropriate, skillful and thoughtful and, yes, his neighbour was called Tom. At the time David was thought to be incapable of such interaction.

There is a warmth of feeling and achievement when, for a 'snap-shot' in time, we as occupational therapists provide the ingredients to enable a person to achieve well-being. We are often asked why we work with people who have dementia, and are often subjected to the statement 'but there's nothing you can do'. We hope we have begun to respond to and challenge these negative views in such a way as to open more possibilities for occupational therapists to be involved in this clinical field. We believe one of the most clearly expressed reasons to maintain current services and pursue new opportunities for involvement in the treatment and rehabilitation of people who have dementia is Agnes' statement: 'I don't know what I did, but boy did I enjoy it'.

References

Allen, C., Earhart, C. and Blue, T. (1992) *Occupational Therapy Goals for the Physically and Cognitively Disabled.* Bethesda, MD: American Occupational Therapy Association Inc.

Kitwood, T. (1997) *Dementia Reconsidered – The Person Comes First.* Buckingham: Open University Press.

Perrin, T. and May, H. (2000) *Wellbeing in Dementia: An Occupational Approach for Therapists and Carers.* Edinburgh: Churchill Livingstone.

Pierce, D. (2001) 'Untangling occupation and activity.' *American Journal of Occupational Therapy 55,* 2, 138–146.

Wey, S. (2000) 'Redefining the possible – Occupational therapy in the treatment of the person experiencing dementia.' Proceedings of OCTEP Clinical Forum, Derby. See www.cot.co.uk/specialist/otop/forums/dementia.php

Yerxa, E. (1967) 'Eleanor Clarke Sagle Lecture. Authentic occupational therapy.' In J. Creek (1999) 'Creative activities.' In 1990 in text *Occupational Therapy in Mental Health.* Edinburgh: Churchill Livingstone.

Further reading

Craig, C. (2002) *Creative Environments: A Practical Approach to Art Activities.* Stirling: Dementia Services Development Centre.

Craig, C. (forthcoming) *Meaningful Making: A Practice Guide for Occupational Therapy Staff.* Stirling: Dementia Services Development Centre.

Killick, J. and Allan, K. (2001) *Communication and the Care of People with Dementia.* Buckingham: Open University Press.

Wood, W. (1998) 'The genius within.' *American Journal of Occupational Therapy 52,* 5, 320–325.

CHAPTER 14

Speech and Language Therapy

Joy Harris

As a speech and language therapist working with people with dementia I would define rehabilitation using terms like enabling, supportive or maintenance as used by Kate Malcomess (2001), which I believe describe more accurately what I do although, as I will describe later in this paper, some of my work aims to be restorative.

Speech and language therapists are concerned with communication in its broadest sense. Through communication, we are able to interact as human beings. It allows us to share experiences, ideas, information, etc. via verbal and nonverbal channels. It is central to our personhood and the effects of impairment on our ability to express ourselves can be all encompassing. It is worth noting that a communication disability is not one person's problem but the problem of anyone who comes into contact with that person. We therefore all have reasons for wanting to bridge that difficulty.

Language breakdown

Dementia affects communication in many ways and language function may be affected:

1. Early stage: Difficulties with semantic function (meaning of words) and pragmatic function (using language appropriately)

2. Moderate stage: Difficulties with syntactic function (grammatical structure)

3. Severe stage: Difficulties with phonemic function (sound system)

However, every person is unique, their levels of impairment will vary and how that impairment impacts on their functioning and general well-being will vary also.

The language breakdown results in the following common features of language difficulties associated with dementia, though it must be stressed that not every person will experience all of these:

- difficulty following a conversation
- slowness at responding
- poor turn-taking in conversation
- no initiation of conversation – only replies when someone else starts it
- conversation wanders with frequent change of topic
- speech is empty, conveys very little information
- difficulty following the television or radio
- failure to appreciate humour or sarcasm (linguistically)
- difficulty remembering names of objects, people or places
- using the wrong word
- frequent repetition of the same phrase or topic
- asks the same question again and again
- mispronounces words
- difficulty understanding written material although may still read aloud
- difficulty writing.

I think it is clear from this list that these symptoms of communication breakdown will markedly affect a person's daily functioning and it is important to note that changes in language, albeit often subtle, are one of the early symptoms of dementia. For this reason, I believe that it is vitally important that communication issues are addressed from the point of diagnosis and that is what we are working towards where I work.

I work with two multidisciplinary teams specializing in dementia care in East Lothian. Core members of the team include the psychiatrist, CPN, social worker, occupational therapist and day hospital charge nurse, whilst a psychologist, liaison nurse (between the service and nursing homes) and I work across both teams. The service comprises a memory clinic for early assessment and diagnosis. Newly diagnosed patients and their carers are allocated a key worker in the dementia team, depending on their specific need, and are invited to attend a rolling six-week programme of information and support. This programme covers information about the East Lothian Dementia Service. The nature of the illness is explained by one of the nurses on the team. Benefits/legal issues are covered by the social worker, and a representative from a local carer support organization explains the advice and support they can offer to family and friends. The next two sessions are talks from a physiotherapist, psychologist, occupational therapist and myself. I use this talk to give general advice about maintaining communication skills, encouraging carers to think about their role in this, and explaining how they can contact me if they want assessment and advice.

When the person is first seen at the memory clinic, they complete a speech and language questionnaire which asks questions about any changes in their communication that they may have noticed and, more specifically, if they are concerned about it. If they indicate concern, they are offered an in-depth assessment. Relatives are asked to complete the same questionnaire and if they indicate concern when their relative does not they are offered information and advice on specific communication strategies.

Those who require full assessment are seen over a period of two to three hour sessions. I use several different assessments, and pick the ones that seem most appropriate to the person when I first meet them. Those most commonly used are the Boston Naming Test, Verbal Fluency Tasks, Cookie Theft Description and Verbal Commands. The Naming Test gives information on the extent of a person's naming deficits and whether they can be cued in easily with either a semantic or phonemic cue. Verbal Fluency Tasks are when the person is asked to name as many items as they can within a category in one minute. People find this progressively more difficult as the dementia develops. Cookie Theft Description is a detailed picture, which the person is asked to describe. What they say is transcribed and the fluency of the language, the relevancy, the attention to detail, the level of repetition, etc. is noted. Verbal Commands are a set of increasingly complex verbal instructions, which the person is asked to do. It gives data on the amount of information a person can process, retain and act on, at any one time. These four tasks give an overall picture of a person's communication strengths and weaknesses. It is often very helpful to do still more detailed assessment but I will only proceed to this if I have established that the person is happy and willing to do more. The assessments I might then use are the Arizona Battery for Communication Disorders in Dementia, RBANS (Repeatable Battery for the Assessment of Psychological Status) or the Barnes Language Assessment.

I believe that people with dementia being actively involved in their assessment and therapy is part of the 'rehab' process and that it should equally involve the closest carer where possible. We have a huge responsibility as professionals to carefully balance our interventions so that expectations are not raised unrealistically and to encourage and empower carers to respond more appropriately without increasing their sense of burden and responsibility. This requires sensitivity on the part of the clinician and careful monitoring of the situation by the team as a whole. I find that people newly diagnosed and in the early stages generally fall into two distinct categories – those who enjoy the assessment process and are keen to discover and discuss the effects of memory on their communication and those who definitely do not want that information. As I have already made clear, the latter group are not further assessed, although they may be happy to engage in therapeutic activities with me.

What do I mean by therapy? Therapy may be seen as beneficial, healing, restorative and I believe that much of what I do as a speech and language therapist should be viewed as a holistic approach to the person and/or carer, and is not confined to remediating specific impairment. Therapy may be direct or indirect, i.e. specifically with the person, or by altering the communication environment or advising carers on specific communication strategies.

Direct therapy varies depending on the individual, but I would like to describe one case of a man with probable vascular dementia. This man had previously run successful businesses and was considered by himself and others to be very capable and articulate prior to the onset of dementia. He was previously a gregarious man and prided himself on his many abilities. Whilst he has found the diagnosis devastating, he is highly motivated to do something that might preserve his abilities.

When I first met him shortly after confirmation of the diagnosis, his expressive problems were probably his most obvious area of difficulty. He is extremely verbose and the meaning of his utterance frequently becomes obscured as he loses the thread. I was immediately struck by the amount of detail he was trying to convey and, taking ideas from a single case study described by Kate Swinburn and Jane Maxim (1996) on a man also with vascular dementia, I embarked on a form of therapy aimed at heightening his self-monitoring skills and reducing his utterances to shorter, more specific phrases. First of all I transcribed a 10-minute monologue he produced when asked to speak about himself. I had hoped to look at this in detail with him, but found that just glancing through it with him meant that he appreciated the amount of 'redundancy' in his speech.

We then set about getting him to produce accurate descriptions of verbal pictures. It took two to three sessions before he began to grasp exactly what I was wanting. Part of this time was taken up with (amicable) arguments with him about what was actually relevant to say for each picture and I began to realize that this style of contradiction or non-acceptance of another's view was very much about how he expressed who he was, and an important part of his communication skills. He has a great sense of humour, and in response to my entreating him to be more economical with words, he signalled that he had zipped his mouth up and stopped speaking altogether.

Gradually he started to produce concise sentences to a specific picture cue. It proved more difficult however to generalize this into ordinary conversation and before we were able to take this further, he had to go away on an extended trip abroad and therapy was suspended. It is my intention to resume therapy when he returns but I do not know how much, if any, ground we will have lost. This is a man who has thoroughly enjoyed the therapy sessions – particularly the brow-beating of his therapist! – and I know that he has benefited from being actively involved in the whole process. I do not think this is a suitable therapy for all people, but I think it is an illustration of a person-centred approach that may be applicable to some people in modified forms.

Rehabilitation also occurs within the group environment. Following on from our Information and Support Group, newly diagnosed people and their carers are invited to attend our Memory and Wellbeing Group which runs for two hours once a week. A multidisciplinary team of occupational therapists, the psychologist and myself staffs the group. The aim of the group is to provide activity, mental stimulation, 'counselling', advice about memory aids and carer support. The first hour of the group usually involves some large group activities, such as relaxation, followed by word games, quizzes, etc. In the second hour, people are offered a choice. Those carers who wish to, spend an hour with me discussing communication issues and strategies. I am loosely following a workshop created by Margaret Metcalfe, Speech and Language Therapist, Nottinghamshire Healthcare NHS Trust and I am indebted to her for sharing it with me. She uses a powerful analogy originally coined by Dawn Brooker, Psychologist, Bradford Dementia Group, about a tennis match, i.e. communication is like a game of tennis, with a message rather than a ball being batted backwards and forwards.

The key points of this for carers are that they have to be a coach rather than being there to win; they need to put the 'ball' where the other can reach; and it is easier to coach some people than others. Consideration needs to be given to 'pre-match preparation' such as minimizing background noise and other distractions; consciously relaxing; remembering it may feel like a first for the other person; and gaining the person's full attention first – by touch, greeting, etc. Strategies to help people 'return a serve':

- Say what you think the other is *feeling*.
- Offer what you think the other wants to say.
- Don't correct mistakes, and avoid confrontation.
- Don't shy away from tears and laughter.
- Little and often is often better.

Strategies for 'reaching their serve':

- Identify the emotion.
- Be open to a range of possibilities, e.g. when they say x they mean y (or z or t).
- Put present and past together to understand the other's reality.

Carers need to be reminded of the concept of a 'long match':

- Keep in peak condition.
- Share activities, not just talking.
- Share memories and encourage reminiscence.
- Celebrate often and aim to have fun.

So far, all the carers have joined this group every week and report that it is very helpful. Everyone else meantime is offered a choice of activities such as painting, discussion group, reminiscence games, dominoes, Scrabble, etc. This group as a whole appears to be very successful and enjoyed by all. We have not had anyone drop out yet, but we are anticipating that as their illness progresses, they will voluntarily leave as it ceases to meet their needs.

The Dementia Service provides day hospital care when there is a need for a more protracted psychiatric assessment or intervention. My colleague who provides a hospital-based service will see individuals for assessment and/or therapy as required, but the overall rehabilitation work is done within groups by the nursing staff. There is also an assessment ward which admits people who already have a diagnosis of dementia but may be experiencing sudden or extreme difficulties which require a change in management. My colleague provides a routine screening of their communication which is used to provide advice and support to staff within the ward and may be helpful in determining future management strategies for the patient. Change in behaviour is a frequent cause of a patient being admitted and it is well recognized that behaviour can be seen as a form of communication. It is therefore vitally important that the speech and language therapist contributes to the process of assessment and management of the patient.

Possibly the most difficult area to promote the concepts of communication and rehabilitation is a continuing care ward. Nursing staff are constantly challenged by the rigorous demands of providing basic care to difficult patients who may be significantly communicatively impaired or even mute. My colleague Claire Black describes one approach for these patients in the next chapter.

I have recently been involved in videoing patients on the continuing care ward to monitor their communication with each other, both verbally and non-verbally. This was a difficult project to set up, with issues around consent to be videoed, but I believe it will be a useful and informative tool in the future. The most striking interchange observed was two patients talking to one another but about totally different subjects. In reality, they were both conducting monologues but they were turn-taking and responding appropriately non-verbally as though it was one cohesive conversation. It did not matter that it was a conversation that went nowhere because both appeared to derive emotional benefit from the exchange. This, I believe, takes us back to the fact that communication allows us to interact as human beings and is central to our personhood.

Through loss, we all redefine ourselves – we are still the unique individual but altered in some ways. Dementia is about losses in many forms, communication being one of them. Perhaps adjusting to and celebrating this new individual is really what rehabilitation is about.

References

Malcomess, K. (2001) 'The Reason for Care.' *RCSLT Bulletin*, 595.

Swinburn, K. and Maxim, J. (1996) 'Multi Infarct Dementia – A Special Case for Treatment?' In K. Bryan and J. Maxim (eds) *Communication Disability and the Psychiatry of Old Age.* London: Whurr Publishers.

CHAPTER 15

Speech and Language Therapy Work in Sonas Groups

Claire Black

In my role as a speech and language therapist on a continuing care ward, it can often be difficult to promote the concept of communication. Patients are often significantly communicatively impaired, some may be mute, and too often these individuals in the later stages of dementia are regarded as a homogeneous group, branded collectively by their apparent inability to communicate. In this situation, the speech and language therapist's role is largely involved with environmental changes, the arrangements of seating to promote socialization, ensuring quiet areas, etc., whilst highlighting the importance of non-verbal and modified communication to nursing staff who are constantly challenged by the rigorous demands of providing care.

Sonas aPc (Threadgold 2002) groups are run regularly on the ward by myself, an occupational therapist assistant and/or ward activities organizer. Sonas is a multi-sensory approach that stimulates the senses and enables communication, thereby improving well-being. It is noticeable that patients talk to each other during the group, even if they mainly ignore each other on the ward. From a professional and personal perspective, I have found working with patients in the later stages of dementia as a facilitator of a Sonas group is an insightful, rewarding and humbling experience. Insightful, as one learns more about the individual participants, rewarding as small but significant gains are made, and humbling in that here are a group of people, so often cut off from opportunities to effect communication (perhaps due to other's attitudes more than the nature of their illness), responding positively when given the chance.

Of course it is impossible to argue how clinically effective this type of therapy is. Working with a client group regressing along a conclusively deteriorating pathway, one does not expect hugely positive steps. Perhaps the best way to illustrate it and to convey what this type of group environment can offer, is by sharing some personal observations of individual patients.

A is a man widely regarded as practically mute. Amiable by appearance, he wears a constant smile on his face, but has always presented as completely unresponsive to all attempts at communication. After a few weeks of attending a group he has been observed mouthing the words to many of the regular songs and will now spontaneously clap along to them too.

B is also for the most part non-verbal, except when exhibiting one of his behavioural outbursts, which are generally accompanied by a variety of loud and clear obscenities. As a member of the group however he appears calm and relaxed. When particular music begins he will waltz around the room, with a partner when offered. Who knows what memories this has evoked? What comes across strikingly though, is an elderly gentleman at peace in his world, a far cry from the often disruptive character whose reputation seems to precede him.

C is a more verbal participant than the previous two. This man has always welcomed a chat when I have encountered him in the ward despite typically never remembering my name or who I am. However, after attending the group for just two weeks he now recognizes and greets me as the 'lady from the peaceful room'.

This I hope conveys something of the essence of our group as a place where patients can relax and be given the opportunity and time to communicate through a variety of modalities. These examples are but a few of the individuals with whom I have been privileged to work. Through them I have learned that the individual personality, inherent in us all, remains even in the later stages of dementia and should be given the opportunity to be expressed and responded to.

Reference

Threadgold, M. (2002) 'Sonas aPc: A new lease of life for some.' *Signpost* 7, 1, 35–37.

CHAPTER 16

Dementia and Rehabilitation: A CPN Perspective

Ken Barlow

Not too many years ago, the likelihood of the words rehabilitation and dementia appearing in the same sentence would have been remote indeed, to some perhaps even an oxymoron. It is therefore a measure of the developments in dementia care that specialisms such as 'rehabilitation' are currently being vigorously explored and undertaken in practice. From a community psychiatric nursing (CPN) perspective there are a number of points which need clarification in order to consider the concept in a broader and more meaningful sense. For example, do we have an agreed and workable definition of the term rehabilitation in the context of dementia care? Even more profoundly, what is a CPN and what roles/duties should they perform? The purpose of this chapter is to raise these issues and others, for debate and consideration rather than to necessarily claim to have all the answers.

Question to pose

CPNs currently stand at a crossroads in their development as a specialist discipline within the profession of nursing. Whilst this is true of CPNs in general psychiatry, it is arguably even more the case for CPNs in dementia care, where a broader model of care based upon a bio-psycho-social approach is increasingly coming to the fore. Is it time to ask CPNs to finally cut the apron strings of psychiatry and forge their own identity? And if so, how might this be achieved, both as a discipline and as individual practitioners? Are there sufficient common core values and beliefs across the wide range of CPN practice in dementia care for the term 'CPN' to be an accepted, generic and recognized term of common understanding?

What of rehabilitation in terms of dementia care? Is it the person being 'rehabilitated', is it the family? Are they being rehabilitated from an 'illness' or a social condition? Is the need, in fact, for rehabilitation of the very culture of care in which dementia care is currently based?

Whatever the conclusions reached, CPNs need to reflect upon such questions and use the answers reached to help inform their practice. These questions are not merely a pseudo-intellectual exercise for academic purposes only. Clarification will lead us to a much firmer basis for practice. Some of the questions have their roots in political, financial and social welfare provision, others in the traditional reluctance of nurses to be self-critical in practice.

Rehabilitation in dementia care signifies a major step in the acceptance of people with dementia as persons first and foremost; people's quality of life *can* improve. Are CPNs in dementia care geared up for this or will they continue to sustain the illness-based, medical model belief that the best to be offered is merely TLC until the bitter end?

Tom Kitwood's benchmark work on 'personhood' (1997a and 1997b) paved the way for major developments in dementia care and in particular rehabilitation of people with dementia. His work has been immensely influential in the field and has at its core, the notion that the person with dementia is a person first, foremost and always. In identifying specific needs of people with dementia (Chapter 5, 1997b), Kitwood lays down the foundation for rehabilitation. The need for inclusion, attachment, comfort, identity and occupation, all centred around the need for *love*, are paramount in understanding a person-centred, needs-based approach to rehabilitation in dementia care. If such needs are met, primary prevention will occur in which the requirement for secondary and tertiary rehabilitation becomes unnecessary.

Naomi Feil's approach of Validation Therapy (1982; 1993) was a move away from concentrating upon cognitive abilities as such, toward the affective domain of feelings, experiences and emotions. These are seen as the real repository of resources to be used in maintaining a sense of 'self'. Cheston and Bender (1999) emphasize the need of people with dementia for security. They suggest that with security, cognitive deficits can be placed in a truer perspective and that feeling safe should, in itself, be a primary aim for all service/care providers.

For CPNs such distinctions are important. It is easy to be railroaded down the specialist practitioner branch line armed with a great deal of information, rating scales and outcome measurements, whilst failing to recognize the intrinsic value of the nurse/client relationship itself. An holistic view of people with dementia is essential. Of course there is evidence of the importance of cognitive rehabilitation (DeVreese *et al.* 2001; Gatz *et al.* 1998), but CPNs need to be attuned to the whole person, not merely their cognitive/functional abilities. Cognitive rehabilitation is a useful therapeutic tool, of which more CPNs should be made aware, but rehabilitation of the person as a whole is more than the sum of their functional parts.

CPNs working in the field of dementia have emerged in parallel to developments in dementia care in general. If dementia care was an abandoned waif taken in by sympathetic general psychiatry, then the psychiatric nurses involved were the well-intentioned, though not particularly well-trained, orderlies. Only in recent years has nursing care in dementia gradually emerged as a specialist discipline in its own right. Pertinent questions remain, however. Upon what, precisely, is good practice based? Where is the evidence for this? Do CPNs have access to well-funded post-registration training thereby allowing them to continue to keep up with contemporary developments? Continued professional development for CPNs in dementia care is essential. To retain credibility in the field CPNs need to assert this right. It could be argued that before we start exploring rehabilitation of others we should be addressing our own professional shortfalls first.

Clarifying the term 'rehabilitation'

Increasingly, and quite rightly, dementia care is being provided through a multi-disciplinary approach. This allows for the utilization of each practitioner's individual skills in providing comprehensive care. The dilemma facing practitioners is establishing precisely what those skills are and how they differ from one discipline to another. There is a grave danger of CPNs, occupational therapists, social workers and others all being reduced to a generic, nondescript 'dementia care worker'. A jack-of-all-trades and master of none. These people will, in higher grades at least, be so busy co-ordinating care provided by others that there will be precious little time left to practise their own unique art.

Such short sightedness could fatally sabotage any attempts at developing the concept of rehabilitation in dementia care. Enabling someone with dementia to recover control, to assert choices and to maintain their sense of individuality cannot be done from a desk shuffling forms around. Rehabilitation is nothing if not about forming personal, one-to-one relationships with people in need and their carers.

When the author first entered psychiatric nursing in the early 1970s care for people with dementia was institutional in nature and setting. Standards were low and expectations limited. Nevertheless the dedication and compassion of a few individuals amidst the lethargy and inertia of the majority stood out. They remain like beacons of light in a mass of best forgotten memories. One of the maxims constantly thrust upon us young tyros when working on the acute admission wards of the time was that 'rehabilitation begins the moment a patient is admitted'. This was preached but only rarely practised and was certainly never mentioned in the context of dementia care.

Now, 30 years later, it is a sign of the progress made in dementia care that the maxim has real relevance. It is the author's contention that rehabilitation of the person might not be necessary if the 'person' is not made a 'patient' in the first place. To this end, the moment someone begins the diagnostic process, their needs as an individual should be established in detail. Respect should be afforded, choices offered, collaborative decisions made and the need for love and security recognized. The person's true sense of self needs to nurtured throughout. Kitwood (1997b) refers to 'Malignant Social Psychology' occurring once people have been diagnosed. The development of early diagnostic services, commonly known as 'memory clinics', has led to the need to guard against malignant social psychology *throughout* the diagnostic process, not merely on formal diagnosis.

CPNs appear in many guises and various locations in dementia care settings. Some are attached to memory clinics. One of the roles of the CPN in such settings should surely be to aim to prevent the need for future rehabilitation by preventing deterioration of the 'self' in the initial stages. Most certainly the CPN's role may be to recommend and implement cognitive training, social interaction strategies, memory enhancement tactics and other approaches, but not to the exclusion of addressing the broader issue of maintaining 'personhood'. Preventative rehabilitation should begin before it is obviously required. It is not about picking up the pieces of a shattered life many months or years down the line.

Tools of rehabilitation

In the experience of the author, one of the most effective tools of rehabilitation, both in terms of prevention and restoration, is Essential Lifestyle Planning (ELP). Sanderson and Smull (2001) have developed this person-centred planning tool with a view to the needs of people with learning difficulties moving from institutional settings to community environments. It is readily adapted to the dementia care field and the author has used it in a number of situations to ensure that a person's stated needs are clearly established at an early stage. This has, in turn, ensured that the person remained paramount. In effect, rehabilitation became unnecessary. The principles involved make it clear that the focus is upon the person. Their idiosyncracies are captured, their likes and dislikes emphasized. Approaches they appreciate are highlighted and those things they value as essential, negotiable or strictly non-negotiable are noted and built into a personal Lifestyle Plan.

Such an approach offers a number of benefits to all concerned. It emphasizes the importance of self and the need to put the person first. In the early stages of dementia it can be the vehicle to establish preferences and wishes for the future. This is particularly important in the light of the Adults With Incapacity (Scotland) Act (2000). It can help establish whether an individual is adapting what Clare (2003) describes as being either a 'self adjusting' or 'self maintaining' strategy in dealing with onset of dementia.

ELP can, where appropriate, form the basis for ongoing care in a variety of settings from homes to hospital or residential care and transfer between the two, should this be necessary. Knowing that someone is frightened of bathing, but enjoys a shower, or prefers male carers for intimate care, or cannot abide being patronized, etc., can help prevent what are often erroneously termed 'challenging behaviours'. Furthermore, such personalized knowledge forces carers to recognize the person as a person and helps ensure this state continues, mitigating against the need for rehabilitation at a later date. It is essential that the Lifestyle Plan is 'alive', not a form hidden in the back of case notes, glanced at briefly on first contact then forgotten about. It needs to be owned by the individual concerned and their immediate carers. It needs to be transferable, and overt in dictating care. Constantly being reviewed and updated, the Lifestyle Plan should be a live and developing process of care reflecting the person's changing needs and preferences. There is little more satisfying than visiting someone at home to find their Lifestyle Plan dog-eared, creased and with various new additions, in different handwriting. This is preventative rehabilitation in action.

ELP is not the only approach that CPNs can use in the rehabilitation process. Many others are available and can often be used in conjunction with each other. Life Story Work, as highlighted by Murphy (1994) and also Gibson (1991), can be therapeutic, enjoyable and stimulating. It can help preserve that sense of self which prevents the loss of identity so characteristic of institutionalization. The restoration of meaning to vague or even lost memories can give colour to a grey life and make the person's life come alive. There are opportunities to involve different generations of family and friends in what is invariably an enriching process for all concerned. Whilst not all memories are necessarily pleasant, Coleman and Mills (1997) suggest that most experienced practitioners find that censorship of repressed or unwanted memories is usually maintained. For many the 'recovery' of a life is synonymous with the recovery of the person.

There are, of course, other therapeutic activities which can help in the process of rehabilitation in dementia. Cognitive Behaviour Therapy (CBT), counselling, procedural memory enhancement and other memory aids are but a few. For CPNs an eclectic view is essential. Underpinning all of these approaches lies the interactional nature of nursing.

Conclusions

CPNs have traditionally had the opportunity to spend quality time with people with dementia and their carers, enabling them to forge that special bond which is almost undefinable in the process of the 'nurse-patient' relationship. Nursing has frequently been described, amongst other things, as 'that which makes the very difficult seem very simple'. Phil Barker (1999) describes nursing as 'neither a science nor an art but is a craft'. He goes on to say that 'Its [nursing] meaning, significance and human value is assigned by the person, family or community who are the recipients of the caring intervention'. This insight may explain why CPNs find it hard to define *how* they do what they do, that magical 'something' which stands them apart from other caring disciplines. It is not for them to define but rather as Phil Barker suggest, it is for others to do so. Whatever conclusion is reached it is clear that CPNs need to retain that crucial, close interactional nursing contact, never more so than in the current climate of change in dementia care.

CPNs, indeed psychiatric nursing in general, stand at a crossroad. As the profession continues to struggle to break free from its medical model background there is a need to establish a role which involves more than becoming mere agents of social control anymore than becoming a generic, one size fits all, care co-ordinator. Contemporary dementia care, and rehabilitation in particular, offers CPNs the opportunity to utilize and develop skills, knowledge and attitudes in order to form ongoing therapeutic relationships with members of a client group increasing in number. CPNs should grasp this opportunity with both hands and all their heart.

Rehabilitation in dementia care can mean different things to different people. The aim should be to prevent institutionalization and depersonalization thereby removing the need for rehabilitation in the first instance. The term 'restoration of the person' may continue to be required as a watchword against complacency. There are tools available with which the maintaining of person-centred values can be integrated into care planning. These are not exclusive to one another but rather can be incorporated on an eclectic, as required, basis.

People with dementia should be as involved in dictating the terms of their care as anyone else. CPNs need to recognize this and value their role as partners in care in preventative rehabilitation in dementia, as in any other nursing setting.

References

Adults with Incapacity (Scotland) Act 2000. Edinburgh: Stationery Office.

Barker, P. (1999) *The Philosophy and Practice of Psychiatric Nursing*. London: Churchill Livingstone.

Cheston, R. and Bender, M. (1999) *Understanding Dementia: The Man with the Worried Eyes.* London: Jessica Kingsley Publishers.

Clare, L. (2003) "'I'm Still Me": Living with the onset of dementia.' *Journal of Dementia Care* March/April, 32–35.

Coleman, P.G. and Mills, M.M. (1997) 'Listening to the Story: Life Review and the Painful Past in Day and Residential Care Settings.' In L. Hunt, M. Marshall and C. Rowlings (eds) *Past Trauma in Late Life: European Perspectives on Therapeutic Work with Older People.* London: Jessica Kingsley Publishers.

De Vreese, L.P., Neri, M., Fiorainti, M., Bellri, L. and Zannetti, O. (2001) 'Memory rehabilitation in Alzheimer's Disease, a review.' *International Journal of Geriatric Psychiatry 16,* 794–809.

Feil, N. (1982) *Validation: The Feil Method.* Cleveland: Edward Feil Productions.

Feil, N. (1993) *The Validation Breakthrough.* Baltimore: Health Promotions Press.

Gatz, M., Fiske, A., Fox, L., Kaskie, B., Kasle-Godley, J.E., McCullum, T.J. and Wetherall, J.L. (1998) 'Empirically validated psychological treatments for older adults.' *Journal of Mental Health and Ageing 4,* 9–45.

Gibson, F. (1991) *The Lost Ones, Recovering the Past to Help the Present.* Stirling: Dementia Services Development Centre.

Kitwood, T. (1997a) 'The experience of dementia.' *Ageing and Mental Health 1,* 13–22.

Kitwood, T. (1997b) *Dementia Reconsidered: The Person Comes First.* Buckingham: Open University Press.

Murphy, C. (1994) *'It Started with a Sea Shell.' Life Story Work and People With Dementia.* Stirling: Dementia Services Development Centre.

Sanderson, H. and Smull, M. (2001) *Essential Lifestyle Planning.* Manchester: North West Training and Development Team.

CHAPTER 17

The Contribution of Social Work to the Rehabilitation of Older People with Dementia: Values in Practice

Maria Parsons

This chapter outlines the unique contribution that social workers make to the rehabilitation of older people with dementia, through the application of distinctive values to roles, tasks and goals, which take into account the progressive nature of the illness whilst enabling service users and carers to achieve optimal health and well-being through working in partnership with other professionals and care staff.

Social workers are usually employed as care managers by local councils with social care responsibilities, often in social services departments, or increasingly in joint health and social care agencies. Together with primary and secondary health services, social services are involved in the delivery of intermediate care services for people who might otherwise face a prolonged and unnecessary stay in hospital, inappropriate admission to acute patient care, long term residential care or continuing NHS in-patient care services. A core activity of intermediate care is the rehabilitation of older people who need a period of recuperation following elective surgery, or who have had an accident or experienced some sort of remediable health crisis.

Since medical science construes dementia as terminal disease, older people affected are deemed to lack potential for rehabilitation. Medically orientated, time limited rehabilitation services that focus on the restoration of functional ability to former levels are therefore usually provided in ways that are incompatible with the needs of older people with dementia, who are effectively excluded from intermediate care and rehabilitation (Herbert 2002). Only 4 per cent (10) of 253 intermediate care projects for older people in south west England were for those with dementia (Social Services Inspectorate and National Health Services Executive South West 2001), whilst less then half of 26 local authorities in the south east of England responding to a survey of services for older people with mental health needs had specialist intermediate care beds, and more than half had intermediate care protocols which debarred older people with dementia (Kerslake, Moultrie and Parsons 2003).

The importance of values in social work

Social work largely rejects the medical model of dementia as a disease state, espousing the view of dementia as a disability that is exacerbated by negative societal attitudes, social behaviour and poor design of physical environments. This perspective is central to professional practice and culture and serves to differentiate it from medicine, nursing or occupational therapy. Encompassing respect for human dignity and worth, integrity and professional competence, social work values resonate strongly with those of person-centred care which provide direction and meaning. Hence social workers are unique amongst other health and care professionals in pursuing social justice through the promotion of citizenship, participation, community presence, equality, anti-oppressive practice and empowerment. In applying such values to action social workers are committed to challenging individuals and social institutions that discriminate against individuals and groups who, because they are old or have dementia, are deemed to be of less worth. In all contact with older people, social workers seek to validate their subjective experience and to counter social exclusion. Importantly, such principles are the basis on which explicitly or implicitly social workers make decisions in respect of ethical dilemmas involving risks to older people with dementia, which are some of the most complex faced by health and care professionals.

Whilst the target for most health interventions is the individual, social work is concerned not only with the person and their subjective experience, but also with relationships between individuals, groups and communities, and the social, cultural and economic processes that influence these in society at large. Thus 'the dementing process should be viewed as the outcome of the dialectical interplay between two tendencies. The first is neurological impairment, which does indeed set the upper limits to how a person can perform. The second is personal psychology an individual has accrued, together with the social environment with which he or she is surrounded (Kitwood and Bredin 1992). In working with older people with dementia, social workers therefore focus on mobilizing resources that can support the restoration of well-being and independent living to an optimum level, particularly in meeting specific needs to do with housing, mobility, income, daily living and occupation. Reframed in this way, rehabilitation is not a discrete post hospital event but rather an ongoing process, which aims to help individuals with dementia maintain a quality of life through the trajectory of changes and losses associated with the illness.

Since social workers are located in community settings as well as hospitals they are in an exceptional position to contribute to positive outcomes for older people with dementia. Most social workers are care managers who are members of generic teams for older people, community-based mental health teams for older people, intermediate care or enablement teams or hospital-based multidisciplinary teams. Core community team members in small locality teams may be social workers and community psychiatric nurses (CPNs) who can nevertheless manage and provide innovatory services as demonstrated by the Bridgend community care teams (Audit Commission 2000). More extensive teams will have social workers, CPNs or district nurses, and occupational therapists (OTs), with input from psychogeriatricians and, depending on availability, other allied health professionals such as physiotherapists, speech and language therapists, health visitors and pharmacists. Some teams for older people such as Milton Keynes Joint Elderly Mental Health Services Team or Kingston on Thames Community Mental Health Team include support workers or care assistants who are involved in providing help for daily living. The Access Team in Suffolk is amongst a number who employ workers seconded from voluntary societies who can offer specialist information, psychosocial support and financial advice to older people with dementia and their carers. Knowsley Community Older Person's Team includes home safety co-ordinators and a well-being project.

Social work roles

There have been significant changes in the traditional roles of social workers following the separation of commissioning services from their provision following the National Health Services and Community Care Act 1990. More latterly, the profession has had to respond to the service integration agenda, and social work is increasingly practised within a healthcare framework, within settings where there is a preponderance of nursing and allied health professionals. For example, psychosocial support and counselling, previously a province of social work, is now undertaken by nurses and allied health professionals who, as in Leeds Community Treatment Team for people with dementia, undertake a wide range of rehabilitation roles.

Assessment

As care managers, social workers have a key role carrying out local authorities' statutory duty to undertake assessments. Sometimes described as 'gate keeping', social workers assess older people with dementia in line with agency criteria, which is used to determine their level of need and to commission services for those deemed to be in priority need. Increasingly, however, CPNs and OTs are also acting as care managers. Research shows differences in both process and outcome between the single assessments of older people carried out by social workers, community nurses and OTs. One study found that social work assessment was person-centred, needs led, reviewed difficulties related to daily living, income, housing, transport, and meeting social and recreational needs, and took account of family support and social networks, whereas OTs focused on functional adjustment and ability, and nurses on health and treatment of illness (Parsons 2001).

These discrepancies should be overcome by the Single Assessment Process, which ushers in validated models of multidisciplinary assessment to reduce duplication and ensure comprehensive coverage. In terms of best practice, a holistic approach to assessment of older people with dementia is likely to be led by a social worker who conducts the initial interview, working jointly with other professionals and drawing on a wide range of disciplinary expertise.

Acting as care managers, social workers are responsible for drawing up individually tailored care plans to promote independence and optimize the quality of life of the person deemed to be in need. This key task involves commissioning and co-ordinating services which meet identified needs. Models of intensive care management whereby social workers have devolved budgets, which enables them to respond to the peaks and troughs in the lives of older people with dementia have been shown to delay institutionalization. Part of their effectiveness is in recognizing that 'rehabilitation' is life long and services are needed to monitor and review service users at regular intervals in order to promote independence and prevent difficulties becoming crises. Good examples include:

- Oxfordshire City and County Age Concern Flexible Carers who provide a befriending service which also enables them to continually monitor the health and well-being of older people with dementia and their carers.

- Poole Dementia Home Care Service, staffed by domiciliary carers given specialist training and linked with the community team.

- Berkshire's St John's Ambulance day centres, which provide seven-days-a-week care.

- Newham day care for Asian elders, which also provides a wide range of other information and advice to services users with dementia.

- Northamptonshire Safe at Home Project which offers aids, adaptations and assistive technology to help support older people and carers remain safely at home. The care manager carries out an assessment and, where needs are identified which might be met by assistive technology, they accompany individuals and carers to a demonstration house where aids and equipment can be tested and selected.

Assessment and support for carers

Social workers have a key role in preventing inappropriate admission to institutional care and promoting safe and timely discharge from hospital through facilitating carers' access to community-based services and resources. In doing so they have to take account of coping strategies that spouses and families develop and try not to undermine carers and pathologize families' best efforts to 'normalize' caring situations that may be challenging and stressful. They are charged with a statutory responsibility to assess the carer's needs even if the person they are caring for does not receive service and in doing so to view carers as partners. However carer's assessments have a low priority in many authorities and, where information is available, low completion rates are reported. Additionally, the quality of assessments is variable and few councils provide a good or adequate range of support services (Audit Commission 2004). Effective models of carer support have been developed by Cornwall Social Services Department and by Bradford Council, with a particular focus on the needs of carers from black and ethnic minorities, but it is clear that service for carers need to be improved.

Social work in hospital

As care managers, social workers are part of multidisciplinary teams involved in assessment, care planning and discharge from hospital. Many older people enter hospital following a crisis, often due to the lack or unavailability of alternative community-based services. Some success has been reported in locating social workers in Accident and Emergency Units or in Medical Assessment Units, where they may be able to identify resources which could lead to a person with dementia not being admitted. Social workers may or may not have contact with older people with dementia, depending on ward staff making referrals, but most hospitals have multidisciplinary assessment teams which seek to identify those people who are likely to have difficulties. However, the volume of demand for long-term placements and support packages for older people, especially those with complex needs, has led to beds being 'blocked'. In response, the Department of Health has produced a helpful specialist discharge planning checklist for people with dementia (Department of Health 2003), but the paucity of suitable placements or resources continues to hinder best practice. The Community Care (Delayed Discharges) Act 2003 is designed to compel local authorities to make more placements available for people coming out of hospital. Social workers may therefore be placed in the invidious position of acting as advocates for older people with dementia (especially where there is no family to do so) who often wish to return home, whilst discharging the local authority's responsibilities to place service users or risk being fined. In Oxfordshire, however, as in many other counties, the results of social work assessments are communicated to the Access and Care teams who decide what services would best meet the identified needs and arrange for these to be made available. Thurrock Community Mental Health Team have developed an effective home from hospital specialist team which enables hospital-based social workers to refer older people with dementia to a specialist team for longer term support.

Conclusions

As a profession, social work does not subscribe to the biomedical view of dementia with its dire consequences for cognitive impairment (Harding and Palfreyman 1997). Its values are congruent with a person-centred approach to practice, and social workers seek to ensure not only that an individual is understood in their social context but that disabilities arising in a world privileging able-bodied people are addressed. Social work roles have shifted almost wholly to care management and a voluminous literature attests to the perceived threats of these changes to social work. Yet in carrying out local authority duties for needs led assessment, commissioning individualized services and the assessment of carers needs, whilst working in multidisciplinary teams, social workers are uniquely placed to contribute a social perspective to complex issues of rights, responsibilities, resources and rationing, all of which are key themes in debates about the rehabilitation of older people with dementia.

References

Audit Commission (2000) *Forget Me Not. Older People with Mental Health Problems*. London: Audit Commission.

Audit Commission (2004) *Support for Carers of Older People*. London: Audit Commission.

Department of Health (2003) *Discharge from Hospital: Getting it Right for People with Dementia.* Department of Health: Health and Social Care Change Agent Team. Available from: www.doh.gov.uk/jointunit/changeagenteam

Herbert, G. (2002) *Exclusivity or Exclusion? Meeting Mental Health Needs in Intermediate Care.* Leeds: Nuffield Institute for Health, Leeds University.

Kerslake, A., Moultrie, K. and Parsons, M. (2003) *The Shape of Future Care for Older People with Mental Health Needs.* Oxford: Oxford Dementia Centre with Friends of the Elderly.

Kitwood, T. and Bredin, K. (1992) 'Towards a theory of dementia care: personhood and well-being.' *Ageing and Society 12,* 269–287.

Parsons, M.S. (2001) *The Quality of Care Management in Hertfordshire Social Services EPD Teams.* Oxford: Oxford Dementia Centre.

Harding, N. and Palfreyman, C. (1997) *The Social Construction of Dementia. Confused Professionals?* London: Jessica Kingsley Publishers.

Social Services Inspectorate and National Health Services Executive South West (2001) *Modernising Services for Older People. A Compendium of Intermediate Care and Other Recent Initiatives in Place or Under Development in the South West.* Issue 2 (August 2001) available at: http://www.doh.gov.uk/swro/olderpeopleservices

PART FOUR
Specific Settings

CHAPTER 18

An Australian Model
of Community Dementia Care

Barry Wiggins and Jenny Fahy

In this chapter we describe how, by following a few simple principles, our model of community dementia care can produce a significant rehabilitative effect in regard to the psychosocial functioning of elderly people who have dementia. Within six to eight weeks our model of care can have a major impact on the lives of people with dementia, and particularly those people with dementia who live alone.

Why the need for a community dementia care model?

Best practice residential care for people with dementia is usually provided in a dementia-specific setting where the service provider is able to apply a model of care tailored to the needs of residents who have a dementing illness. Community care in Australia has been primarily focused on supporting people who are elderly and frail, and the range of standard interventions has been suited to supporting people with physical limitations: interventions like providing help with showering, dressing, house cleaning, shopping and provision of meals. This care also tends to be very much task focused.

The problem is that people with dementia who are assessed as being appropriate for a community care service are not necessarily frail. While they may have health issues that need to be managed, other issues such as their confusion, their impaired judgment and their impaired interpersonal skills are the major risk factors in their lives. A task-focused community care service is rarely effective in supporting people with dementia. Instead, these people need a style of service that is client-focused and flexible enough to respond to and compensate for the cognitive dysfunction that dementia causes.

The service model we will describe is one whereby the one service addresses all the identified needs of the client, and there is no health/social work split in terms of service delivery. It is the role of our service to provide whatever it takes to support the client. A registered nurse coordinates the service, but the model is more a social support model than a medical model. If health services such as community mental health teams are used, it is mostly on a consultancy basis, providing advice and support to our service coordinator.

The Hammond Care Group established this model of care in late 1998 on the New South Wales Central Coast, approximately 80 km north of Sydney. The area had a significant shortage of residential aged care accommodation, and the vast majority of the people referred to our service have been people living alone, often without any family living in the district. The service model, supporting just 30 clients in its first year, had the effect of a pilot program in that it demonstrated that many people with dementia can be effectively supported in the community with a quality of life that is at least the equal of what they would experience in residential care. As a result, the Hammond Care Group has attracted additional Commonwealth Government funding that has allowed us to substantially expand the Central Coast service, and to replicate the model of care in four other areas, to the point where we now support 296 people in total.

A typical client profile

A typical client is someone who has been living alone, and who has become increasingly socially dysfunctional in the period before they were referred. Most clients have not been eating well, and are malnourished. They might have also had recent weight loss, giddiness or other complications. And we know that an inadequate diet can exacerbate the effects of dementia. Prior to coming on the program our community dementia care clients have usually been taking prescribed medications in a somewhat reckless or random manner, wavering between under-medicating and over-medicating. They often have very few supportive social networks, and because of their dementia they need practical support more than ever. They might be neglecting their personal hygiene. They may not be washing their clothes – perhaps because they have forgotten how to use the washing machine, but perhaps because they just don't notice that their clothes are dirty. They are probably not managing the finances of the household, and may be forgetting to pay bills or be losing track of where their money is going. It is possible that they are being abused financially, perhaps by unscrupulous tradesmen or by neighbours. With these things going on, it is very unlikely that they are coping very well on an emotional level. They have usually had fewer and fewer appropriate or successful social interactions lately.

Given that they are having practical difficulties in many aspects of their day-to-day lives, they are likely to be worried and agitated or depressed and withdrawn. In more severe scenarios, they may have developed quite paranoid delusions – they may not be eating because they are convinced someone is trying to poison them or they may be in conflict with a neighbour and be convinced that the neighbours are plotting against them. Their neighbours usually have no understanding of what is happening for the person who is our client, and often they just see them as being a nuisance or a threat, as someone who is either mad or dangerous.

Three key factors

There are three key factors in this typical scenario described above, of a person with dementia, living alone, without effective community support:

1. Inadequate diet.

2. Poor medication management.

3. Lack of social and practical support.

Our model sets out to address these three key areas of diet, medication management, and social and practical support. We find that, when we address those three key areas, usually within six to eight weeks there is a marked change in our clients' behaviour and their mental state. The biggest change is that our typical client will no longer be withdrawn, but instead will be trusting of our staff, which allows us to build relationships and be able to help them to engage more fully with the wider community.

Two phases of intervention

Phase one: The first six to eight weeks

In this initial phase we aim to:

- Win a level of baseline trust, so that the client will comfortably allow us into their homes instead of being suspicious of us. Sometimes it takes weeks of visits, where we are just chatting at the front door, before we are allowed into the house. Our staff need a mixture of skill, charm, and perseverance as they try to find ways to engage the client at that stage.

- Improve the client's diet, so that the effects of a previously deficient diet are corrected.

- Organize whatever medication that the client needs to be taking in a way that is as simple as possible, and that allows us to track compliance.

- Identify the safety or risk factors relevant to each individual living in the community, and be able to anticipate the problems that might arise, and how they might be addressed.

- Ensure that the client has practical help to manage the household finances and pay whatever bills that come due. This often means that we need to arrange for them to have a financial guardian appointed, to ensure that they are not being financially exploited.

- Communicate with our clients on an emotional level – we try to communicate a strong sense of support for them and respect for them so that they experience a sense of support.

Since it is so important to have the right staff, we carefully recruit all our own staff: staff who like elderly people, who enjoy a degree of responsibility and who are problem-solvers. We do not broker staff from other services. We build trust by using only two staff, who have regular, consistent contact with the client on different days throughout the week. We also provide a 24-hour, 7-day-a-week on-call telephone support service. For clients who are inclined to become anxious, we leave reminders for them that they can ring our on-call service, and be reassured that our staff are coming, and that people are looking after their interests.

After that initial period of six to eight weeks, we would expect that the client was eating an adequate diet, that their medication was being managed, and that there was a level of trust between our staff and the client. We would expect that the client was feeling safer and more emotionally secure.

Phase two: Consolidation and socialisation

In phase two, our focus is on the following aims:

- Maintenance and consolidation of the plan of support – we want to maintain and consolidate the plan that has the client eating properly, that has them taking medication appropriately, and that is providing them with assistance in managing the household and paying the bills.

- Improving the client's quality of life – by involving them in activities and interactions that have significance and meaning for them – usually related to things they enjoyed, or found meaningful, before the onset of dementia. If we neglect this element then we are not providing any sort of 'holistic' care, but instead simply providing service inputs.

- Addressing and resolving issues of concern – we need to be addressing such issues of concern as they arise, and particularly as the dementing process progresses. Most of our clients have lived in their homes for many years, and their home is the place where they feel safest. Nonetheless, we need to continually assess both the extent to which it is safe for the client to be home, and the extent to which the client is able to enjoy a better quality of life than they might expect if they were in residential care.

Staff with a client-focused, 'can do' attitude

Our model of care tries to identify, and compensate for, the range of risk factors in our client's lives: we try to bring a 'can do' and 'whatever it takes' approach to addressing such issues. If we are to be effective, we cannot operate off a set menu of services but, instead, we need to work out whatever it takes to address these risk factors for each of our clients.

For example, the traditional solution to people not eating well is to organize meals on wheels or an alternative meal service. However, this solution usually does not work with people with dementia, as they tend to not eat the delivered meals. Instead they put meals in cupboards and forget them; they feed them to the dog; they throw them out. So, if the client is to eat properly, we need to come at the issue of food in a different way. That might mean that someone has to be with the client at lunchtime. We might have to cook the meal or re-heat the meal that they are to eat; we might have to set the table and create some atmosphere that is conducive to enjoying a meal and our care worker might have to eat a meal with the client. There is usually more a sense of occasion when we share a meal with someone else. Then we usually need to leave a range of finger food in the house so that our clients are getting food at other times of the day. This also allows us to monitor the amount of food our clients are eating.

We also need to see that the people who are our clients have a quality of life. It is not good enough for people to be simply surviving. There may continue to be areas of their lives that are a struggle but it is crucial that we can help people to get some active enjoyment back into their lives. So our staff spend a lot of time supporting people to do just that: to enjoy life.

Client A

Mr M is 73 years old and lives alone in his own home. His daughter lives close by and supports him. He has profound word-finding difficulties and his language is fragmented. He is disoriented in time and place and on assessment for our service he had a mini-mental score of 8/30. He had also had a large weight loss during the year previous to coming on the program. Mr M's situation came to a head when he lost his driving licence, but continued to drive his car to go to a local social club. His daughter had a young family and was unable to provide him with adequate support, and she was becoming quite stressed as a result.

When we started the service, Mr M was very suspicious of any one coming into his home and was reluctant to accept our support. Our initial focus was on the following issues:

- nutritional support to address the weight loss issue
- medication management
- socialization
- seeing that he stopped driving.

A staff member visited Mr M once a day, usually for an hour, but for longer if Mr M wanted to do his shopping or go to the club for lunch. His daughter had contact on the other two days when our staff did not visit.

Progress in developing a relationship of trust with the client was initially slower than we would have hoped, but after two months we had made good progress. He was by then eating regular meals and had gained weight. We managed to involve him in the preparation of these meals, and he enjoyed helping like this. He had been a keen gardener, and is now taking a very active interest in his garden. He visits the local plant nursery with our staff, and they regularly spend time working with him in his garden. Mr M has also begun to take a very keen interest in his home and we have helped him to begin to paint the woodwork and the outside decking.

Mr M enjoys an outing to the local club once a week to have lunch with the care staff. After we had been able to build some trust, and involve the client in some activities that he enjoyed, the family felt comfortable to remove the car, and therefore prevent him driving. He has now adjusted well to not driving and the care staff and his daughter provide transport when he needs it.

Mr M has now been on the program for 15 months, and our staff have been able to help compensate for some of his cognitive deficits, so that he can continue to interact effectively in the world outside his home (shopping, going out for lunch) and to enjoy those things around the home (painting, gardening) that he had presumably always enjoyed.

Client B

Mrs B is 83 years old and lives alone in a unit within a retirement complex. Her nephew and niece live locally and offer her some support. On assessment for this service, Mrs B was described as being suspicious and at times verbally aggressive, and she had no insight into her cognitive deficits. She was also at risk of malnutrition and was at times confused due to erratic medication administration. Carer stress was an issue for Mrs B's niece because she was concerned that Mrs B was not taking her medication. The niece was not able to see her aunt on a daily basis, and realised she needed more regular contact than she could provide.

A plan was established to address the issues of medication management and nutrition support as well as companionship. A visit seven days a week was established to administer medications as well as to attend to meal preparation. Her niece visited on weekends to assist with these issues, and we kept in close contact in monitoring progress. When our staff started visiting Mrs B she was suspicious at times, and angry that her family had arranged for people to come into her home. The staff had to adopt a very slow and gentle approach, and they spent several visits just chatting with the client, rather than trying to provide any help. During this time they discovered her likes and dislikes in regard to food. They discovered that she enjoyed homemade cookies, so one of the care staff baked a batch for her and this helped to win her over to comfortably allow the staff in her home.

Mrs B has had this support for nine months now, and during this time her nutritional state has greatly improved and she has gained weight. She has had a recent admission to hospital with some gastrointestinal problems but she has since returned home again. Mrs B is very keen to remain in her own home and her family wants to support her to do so. Our staff continue to visit Mrs B daily and they are now very welcome.

Client C

Mrs C is not any particular individual, but is instead typical of many clients, who love to go shopping. One day a week our staff take her grocery shopping at a local shopping mall, and as part of the day they have morning tea or lunch at a coffee shop. It is a highlight of Mrs C's week. However, it is not uncommon for Mrs C to be confused about what day of the week it is, and she quite often rings the on-call coordinator to check if it is shopping day, seemingly hoping it is. Our care workers have often arrived at her house on other days of the week to find her on the front verandah, all dressed up, her bag over her shoulder, and very much looking forward to going shopping that day. For our care worker staff to simply tell Mrs C that she is confused and that it is not her shopping day is normally counter productive. She gets upset and agitated, and we usually cannot distract her from her fixation on wanting to go shopping. If we operated a task-focused service we would continue to try to do whatever house cleaning or other personal care tasks we might have planned to do that day. The result would inevitably be that we would leave her in an agitated and distressed state. This level of agitation and distress would very likely increase after the staff left, leaving the person with dementia less capable and functional than when our staff first arrived. So it is very important that we avoid this outcome.

Instead, we expect our staff to be flexible enough to respond creatively to the client's needs and her most immediate need on such occasions is to go out. Often our staff simply take her shopping that day, and ring in to our office for help in rearranging their visits to other clients. And they put off to later in the week whatever it was that they had originally planned to do with Mrs C that day. At other times our staff will be able to negotiate with Mrs C to take her to the same shopping mall and have coffee with her, but not do the shopping. That means that they don't have to rearrange all their other client visits that day, but it also means the house cleaning has to wait a day or two. Whatever they do, we want our staff to focus on the person, not the task. The outcome of this response is that we leave Mrs C feeling relatively peaceful on such days, after having helped her to experience something she really enjoys, rather than leaving her in an agitated state as would have happened if we had been task focused.

Conclusions

We are able to apply this model of care to effectively support people with dementia in the community, many of whom would otherwise need to be in residential care. This model of dementia community care allows us to have a significant 'rehabilitative' impact in our clients' lives within the space of six to eight weeks by focusing on providing an adequate diet, appropriate medication management and compensating for a lack of social and practical support. We can usually support our clients for an average of approximately two years, and we have been able to support some people for up to four years.

This model of care demonstrates that by being client-focused and flexible, rather than task-focused, we can be very effective in supporting people with dementia to remain at home with a good quality of life. The concepts are simple, rather than complicated or sophisticated. However, there are management and organizational challenges. The recruitment, training and support of staff, and the day-to-day coordination of this type of flexible care need to be well managed, but the results are well worth the additional organizational effort required.

CHAPTER 19

The Central Aberdeenshire Experience

Carolyn Marshall, with case profiles by Allison Black

Our interpretation of rehabilitation

The conceptual framework of rehabilitation of people with dementia is translated into practice in the context of the Central Aberdeenshire Community Dementia Team. The aim of the Team is to ensure that people with dementia and those that care for them receive services that are co-ordinated to meet their needs and help to maintain their quality of life at the highest level possible. These aims are at the heart of the work that we do to empower and support people with dementia to maintain their independence and maximize their quality of life.

The team

We are a multi-disciplinary Team that provides a psychiatric, social work, nursing liaison and care management service to people with dementia and their families and carers. It is jointly funded by Grampian Primary Health Care Trust and Aberdeenshire Council Social Work Service and consists of a consultant old age psychiatrist, a co-ordinator who is a senior social worker, two full time social worker/care managers, three half-time social worker/care managers, 1½ 'G' grade community nurses, a support worker supervisor and team of support workers, and 1½ admin support workers. The Team is in fact two 'sister' teams based in the community hospitals in Huntly and Inverurie and serves a predominantly rural area with four main towns, the largest with a population of approximately 10,000 and a high number of smaller villages and settlements. It was first established in 1989 to provide a community team approach to services for people with dementia in the Inverurie and surrounding area.

The way we work

In 1995 the service was extended to the whole of what is now Central Aberdeenshire when the Team took on a care management function as defined by the NHS and Community Care Act 1990. This, in practice, has enabled the Team to purchase services using community care budgets that are devolved to the individual social workers and nurses. Although the nurses are employed by the NHS Primary Care Trust they have taken on the care management aspect as an integral part of their role within the Team in the same way as the social workers. They have their own care management budgets and also use the social work service's recording systems. This means that both social workers and nurses are responsible for assessing the needs of those referred to the Team and are able to set up imaginative packages of care that are tailored to the individual's needs. In the same way, social workers will offer advice and guidance on dementia and its management to individuals and their carers. Both social workers and nurses perform cognitive functioning tests as part of their overall assessment and liaise closely with the consultant psychiatrist, GPs and other health care and social work staff in the process of determining and meeting the individuals needs.

The nurses and social workers also play a central role in providing training on dementia, service development and carer support. Although the nurses may become involved with those who are less physically able, most of the inter-disciplinary expertise is shared within the Team. This allows the Team to offer a 'one-stop shop' approach to our service users: assessing their needs, purchasing care and providing services such as support groups, advice, guidance and education, and to act as a focal point for liaising with other service providers with and on behalf of those referred to the Team. The person with dementia and their needs are thus kept at the centre of the Team's activities to ensure a seamless service is provided promptly, appropriately and to a high standard.

The Community Dementia Team offers an open referral system and therefore draws its referrals from a wide range of services including community nurses, hospital staff, other social work services, carers and family members, as well as the more traditional means of referral from community psychiatric nurses and psychiatrists. Our main criterion for appropriate referral is that there is a documented diagnosis of dementia made by a psychiatrist or a GP. If the referral is from a non-medical source we would offer advice to the referrer to enable speedy diagnosis. Alternatively, the Team members will make a direct referral to the consultant psychiatrist for psychiatric assessment should they feel it is necessary in the process of carrying out their assessment of need.

The Team has a close working relationship with the consultant psychiatrist for Central Aberdeenshire. There are weekly meetings to discuss concerns in relation to individuals to share assessments and request psychiatric support or review. In this way we can assure a rapid response to concerns in relation to the changing needs of our service users. We have access to assessment beds in the two wards for people with dementia in the community hospitals in Inverurie and Huntly, which allows us to have individuals directly admitted for assessment on a planned basis or, more often, in a crisis.

Using relationships in rehabilitation

The Team also provides services in the form of our support workers. These are our own team of specialist support carers who perform a versatile and flexible role which may put the care manager's care plans into action. They may provide home-based respite, social stimulation or give emotional support to carers and individuals with dementia. They also run small groups that focus on shared interests of individuals in a particular area, and also act as the 'eyes and ears' of the care manager: monitoring and reporting regularly on any changes or concerns. Rather than being task-centred, the cornerstone of the work of the support staff is the development of a trusting relationship with the service users.

This definition and description of the Team and, in particular, of the support work of the Team, hides as wide a variety of activities as is the individuality of the people with whom we work. How the Team works to support people with dementia to maintain their independence and promote a high quality of life is best demonstrated by examples of our practice. Names and identifying situations have been changed to maintain the individual's confidentiality.

Miss Smith

Miss Smith became known to the service some five years ago. She had had a fall at home, was admitted to Accident & Emergency and transferred to the local hospital. Whilst in hospital it became evident that she was disorientated with regard to time. She was referred to the Team for assessment. It was suggested that she be assessed by the consultant psychiatrist as she had had previous contact with psychiatric services. Her relative and main carer described a five-year history of memory deterioration and there were concerns about dietary intake and social isolation as, other than her relative, Miss Smith had no social contacts.

Miss Smith was allocated to the nurse care manager who liaised with the ward staff and the consultant at ward meetings, and with Miss Smith's relative in order to assess her needs and prepare a care plan. Because of her memory problems at that stage, Miss Smith had no awareness of her need for support and there were concerns about whether she would agree to the care. The consultant psychiatrist painted a gloomy picture and was reluctant to condone her return to the community. However, her relative was keen that she remain at home as long as possible, as she knew that would be Miss Smith's wish. The nurse care manager agreed that she should be given the opportunity to try out support at home in an attempt to achieve a healthier diet and reduce her social isolation. Both the care manager and Miss Smith's relative knew that this would be challenging.

The nurse care manager arranged for a private agency to provide three daily visits, to prepare meals but the services were refused; Miss Smith would either refuse to answer the door or not permit the carer over the threshold. The private agency was withdrawn and the nurse care manager continued to visit and monitor the situation for some time until she felt it was appropriate to reintroduce care. In consultation with Miss Smith, her relative and the support worker supervisor, a plan was prepared to gradually introduce support workers. It was acknowledged that the plan might take some time to have any degree of success.

At first the carers were to provide mealtime visits, but were only able to engage with Miss Smith either on the doorstep or by having a chat through the window. Gradually, over time, as she became accustomed to their visits and their relationship developed, she began to let the workers into the house for a chat, or agreed to go out for a walk with them. The support workers gave regular reports to the care manager, and expressed some concerns regarding her continuing poor diet and self care.

The nurse care manager reassessed the situation and felt that the support should continue. Over time she began to go out in the car with the support worker and they would drop in at the local day centre where she enjoyed the company and food that was on offer. When the offer was made for her to attend the centre Miss Smith gladly agreed, and now attends three days a week where she enjoys good food and a range of social activities and friendship. The support worker visits when she is not at day care when they take her shopping, prepare a snack or take her out for a meal. They also take her to the hairdresser and manicurist on a regular basis and she permits them to help with some personal hygiene. Miss Smith has developed a good relationship with her support workers and now enjoys their company. Regular contact is maintained with her relative who will make suggestions to the support workers about her care needs and they will attempt to act at Miss Smith's own pace.

In this way she has remained in control of her life whilst her support has enabled her to remain independent and has revitalized her social life.

Mrs Brown

Mrs Brown was referred to the Team four years ago. She had no living relatives and also lived a very isolated life. She was aware that her memory was deteriorating but there was no diagnosis at this point. The social worker/care manager in the Team liaised with the GP to arrange for psychiatric assessment and it was agreed that she would make the referral at our weekly meeting to speed up the process. The consultant and the social worker arranged to visit jointly so that possible services could be discussed at the same time. The consultant diagnosed Alzheimer's disease and this was discussed and explained to Mrs Brown. Her main needs at that point were for some social stimulation and she agreed to attend the local day centre.

Later that year Mrs Brown had a fall. The social worker maintained contact when she was in hospital and arranged for local authority homecare to help with some personal care when she was discharged. It became evident that she was having difficulty coping with her day-to-day activities: bills were unpaid, the phone was cut off, she was failing to attend day care, her personal hygiene and home environment were deteriorating.

The Dementia Team support worker was introduced to supplement homecare visits. Initially this was a befriending visit to get to know Mrs Brown and what she enjoyed doing. Gradually, as she developed a relationship, the support worker would take her out for lunch and reintroduced her after lunch brandy, which Mrs Brown said she used to enjoy. The support worker also identified problems that were inhibiting her mobility. She fed this back to the social worker/care manager for aids to help her to move more freely around her home. Mrs Brown's insight remains good and she expressed a wish to redecorate her house. Supported by the care manager and with Mrs Brown's permission, the support worker discussed the financial aspects of refurbishing her house with her financial adviser. She arranged for the house to be redecorated and helped Mrs Brown buy new furniture and carpets. She liaised with the occupational therapist to have a disabled shower fitted, appropriate locks fitted to doors and outdoor steps made safe. This was all carried out while fully involving Mrs Brown, and she has enjoyed shopping for new items for her house.

The support worker also helps with regular trips to the chiropodist, hairdresser, GP and for shopping. Two years ago she expressed a wish to go on holiday as she used to enjoy trips abroad before her health deteriorated. In consultation with her financial adviser, the support worker and Mrs Brown discussed and planned a holiday. Mrs Brown requested that the support worker accompany her as she knew she could not manage on her own. Arrangements were made to allow this to happen and proved to be very successful, so that it has become an annual event. The support worker has now started life story work with Mrs Brown and is trying to find some of her old friends in the area with a view to re-establishing contact.

CHAPTER 20

Rehabilitation in Acute Medical Settings: A Nursing Perspective

Sarah Rhynas

Introduction

Rehabilitation is an integral part of every nurse's work. Some might suggest that rehabilitation and the promotion of independence are definitive aspects of nursing. Virginia Henderson in her influential definition of nursing suggested that nurses should 'assist the individual, sick or well, in the performance of those activities contributing to health or its recovery (or to a peaceful death) that he would perform unaided if he had the necessary strength, skill or knowledge and to do this in such a way as to help him gain independence as soon as possible' (Henderson 1966). Since this definition was written in the 1960s healthcare and society more generally have undergone major changes and services have been developed in response to medical and technological advance, the rise in the disability movement and the growing financial crisis in health care. Rehabilitation has become central to health care provision and specialist rehabilitation nurses have been employed in areas as diverse as orthopaedics, cardiac care, head injuries, mental health and more recently in elderly care. However, rehabilitation remains the responsibility of nurses in general ward areas as well as those practising in specialist units. This chapter will focus on the role of the nurse in rehabilitation of people who have dementia in the general ward setting. It will consider the skills involved in rehabilitation nursing and will discuss the conceptual, practical and ethical challenges of rehabilitating people with dementia in an acute hospital setting.

Rehabilitation nursing

Much of the literature on rehabilitation considers care in specialist units. This literature suggests that public attitudes and expectations have changed as technological improvements and advancing medical treatments allow larger numbers of people to survive illness and accidents (Livingstone 1991; Meyer 1993). Expectations of old age have also changed as people live longer and lead more active lives well into their advancing years. Rehabilitation has become an important part of the care of older people as they seek to maximize their functional abilities and retain their independence. People living with dementia are an increasingly significant group within the elderly population. The specific rehabilitation needs of this group must be recognized if nurses are to provide high quality care to this group of patients.

While the specialist elderly rehabilitation centres are hugely important in the successful rehabilitation of many elderly people, it is important to recognize that resources are stretched and specialist services are not available to all those who may benefit from them. Nurses on general wards play an important and often unrecognized part in the rehabilitation of older people, particularly in the early days of the hospital admission. This may be particularly true of patients who have dementia, as they may recover from the acute phase of illness more slowly or may not always be admitted to specialist rehabilitation areas.

In order to be successful in the rehabilitation of those who have dementia, nurses must develop certain key skills. Keen assessment skills, abilities in teaching and motivating patients and a willingness to work in a multidisciplinary team are vitally important skills in rehabilitation (Meyer 1993). In the acute medical setting all of these skills are important in determining the outcome of an individual patient's rehabilitation. Referrals to physiotherapists and occupational therapists are often made through the nursing staff. A thorough and accurate nursing assessment can, therefore, be influential in determining the starting point of the rehabilitation process. Nursing staff often spend longer periods of time with patients than other members of the multidisciplinary team. It is, therefore, important that the nursing staff collaborate closely with therapy staff in order to reinforce the messages being given during the therapy sessions. This is particularly important when caring for a person who has dementia, as more reinforcement may be necessary and benefit can be gained from practising skills and techniques on a regular basis.

Challenges in the nursing rehabilitation of people with dementia

Rehabilitation is as much a philosophy as it is considered to be a particular area of care or nursing practice (Preston 1994). In specialist rehabilitation units this philosophy underpins the structures and routines of the setting, promoting patient independence in every area of daily life. In the acute hospital setting rehabilitation is only one among many conflicting priorities that shape the routine of the care setting. Rehabilitation challenges the general ward nurse at a variety of levels. It raises a number of conceptual, practical and ethical challenges for nurses working in acute medicine. These issues will now be discussed in more detail.

Conceptual challenges

Rehabilitation of the person with dementia can be conceptually challenging. Rehabilitation challenges the nurse in his or her thinking about dementia and the course of dementing illness. Those living with dementia are often thought to have poor rehabilitation potential and can be placed lower in the priority list for specialist rehabilitation beds. Research has shown that there can be considerable benefit in rehabilitation for those who live with dementia (Diamond *et al.* 1996; Goldstein *et al.* 1997), refuting the notion that specialist services are of less value to this group of patients. Functional abilities can be improved along with coping strategies and subsequently there can be huge benefits in terms of confidence, willingness to maintain social contacts and ability to pursue personal goals. While there is considerable evidence to indicate the value of rehabilitation in people with dementia, the nature of the discussions between members of the multidisciplinary team highlights a broader and more complex issue about how dementia is conceptualized by professional carers.

The way in which dementia is understood by professional carers can be hugely influential. There is considerable evidence to suggest that the way in which dementia is understood may influence an individual's behaviour and inter-action with the person who has dementia (Sabat 1998). Behaviours and levels of disability demonstrated by people who have dementia have been found to be related to the interaction of dementia suffers with others in society (Sabat 1994; Vittoria 1999; Wood and Ryan 1991). Therefore the extent to which the person with dementia progresses positively with their rehabilitation is influenced by the nature and quality of the interaction between nurse and patient. Little work has been done on how nurses conceptualize dementia but education, socialization, structures and attitudes are all thought to effect the conceptualization process (Asch 1946). Most nurse education focuses on a medical model of health and ill-ness which highlights the symptoms and care issues raised by dementing illness. Dementia-specific education tends to be limited within the course of pre-regis-tration nurse education and so nurses may lack an overview of the course of dementia or of the more positive and less problem-focused dementia literatures. Nurses' understandings of dementia may, therefore, be shaped by biomedical literature and the structures of acute medical care settings. These influences may in turn cause acute sector nurses to interact with people who have dementia in specific ways, perhaps focusing on functional deficits and symptoms rather than prioritizing social and psychological adjustments.

Rehabilitation literature highlights the importance of psychological support of the patient and realistic goal setting in achieving the rehabilitation aims. Adjusting to changes in body image or functional abilities is an important part of the rehabilitation process (Meyer 1993). Much of the rehabilitation literature concentrates on rehabilitation after a specific change of health state or dramatic event or accident. The onset of dementia is likely to be insidious and the realisation of cognitive decline gradual. This process has the potential for far reaching psychological effects undermining the confidence of the individual. The ward nurse has an important role, offering sensitive and realistic support to patients who have dementia. This may be an area of rehabilitation that is neglected by nurses in the acute sector who tend to focus on functional aspects of rehabilitation. However, nurses spend a great deal of time with patients over the course of a day and may be well placed to offer the vital support and encouragement needed to improve the rehabilitation of people with dementia in the acute hospital ward. This is an area that could be highlighted through education of acute sector nurses and improved as awareness of dementia specific issues is raised.

Further conceptual challenges arise in the acute sector because of the mixed aetiology of dementia evident in this setting. Many patients suffer from drug and alcohol-induced dementia which may raise specific challenges for nurses. Many of these patients are younger which may change the presentation. For example, lifespan issues may be different with less evidence of continuous decline in cognitive function and more examples of relapses and repeated admissions to hospital. This pattern can be challenging for nursing staff who have to remain highly motivated in order to repeatedly support the rehabilitation of this group of patients.

Dementia has been described as a social death (Cohen and Eisdorfer 2002). This is only one conceptualization of dementia but it raises important issues about the kind of rehabilitation and support that may be appropriate for nurses to provide in the acute hospital sector. Nursing assessment and care planning can be very functionally focused. It is, therefore, vitally important that those nurses involved in the rehabilitation of people who have dementia take full account of the social rehabilitation required. People who have dementia may need support in order to regain confidence in social situations and to continue to interact within the social world that they live in. This may mean that considerable time and effort needs to be spent on making sure that the person feels comfortable with coping strategies and is aware of where support can be found if it is required. Nurses have an important role to play in this social rehabilitation. It may often be the ward nurse, in collaboration with multidisciplinary colleagues, who sets up support for the individual when they are discharged from hospital. The importance of this discharge planning can not be underestimated as the instigation of effective support may be important in improving quality of life for the person and preventing a readmission to hospital.

Nurses' conceptualization of dementia may be influential in determining the nature and quality of their interaction with dementia patients and the subsequent success of the rehabilitation process. Much nurse education concentrates on a medical model of dementia and this can lead to a focus on functional aspects of assessment and rehabilitation. It is important that nurses fully understand the importance of social and psychological support in the rehabilitation of dementia patients. Even in busy acute medicine wards, nurses spend significant amounts of time with patients and have the potential to support and develop the abilities of patients in their care.

Practical challenges

Having discussed some of the conceptual challenges for nurses in rehabilitating dementia patients in acute settings, it is important now to turn to some of the practical challenges. Nurses in acute wards have a wide variety of demands on their time. Medical emergencies take priority and this leads to a situation where rehabilitation can be seen as a secondary concern. Despite this major difficulty, nurses in acute medical areas can work with patients, sometimes over extended periods of time, to develop their skills and support active rehabilitation.

The acute ward environment is not conducive to a rehabilitative approach to care. The ward can be a busy and noisy area where there can be lots of distractions for those who may have trouble focusing on a specific task. Patient turnover is usually fast and beds are often moved in order to deal effectively with acutely unwell patients. Reinforcement of skills and ongoing support of a dementia patient who is having rehabilitation can be a real challenge in this setting. The nursing staff too may need support to develop skills both in rehabilitation and in specific dementia-related issues. General rehabilitation and the promotion of independence is part of the remit of any practising nurse. However, the skills involved in working with people who have dementia may need to be developed and education may be required in order that goal setting and care planning for people with dementia is realistic and takes account of the course of dementia.

Ethical challenges

Rehabilitation of dementia patients also raises ethical challenges for nurses. In busy acute medical settings nurses have to prioritize and make decisions about how best to manage their workload. The structures of the environment may all add to this dilemma, as pressure on beds requires that nurses work with those who are close to discharge at the expense of those who require more time-intensive intervention.

The shortage of specialist rehabilitation beds often leads healthcare teams to discuss the potential of different patients to benefit from the intensive rehabilitation placements. Nurses and other members of the multidisciplinary team are heard to discuss patients in terms of how 'rehabable' they might be. The potential for people with dementia to benefit from rehabilitation has been established, however, this ethical dilemma continues to challenge nurses in the acute sector.

Nurses in the acute sector also feel somewhat unprepared for a role in rehabilitation for those who have dementia. Dementia itself can be seen as a challenge to the identity of the nurse as it crosses some of the boundaries between mental health and general nursing specialities (Watson 1997). This can become an issue for nurses when they are discussing future needs with a person who has dementia and their family while feeling unprepared for this task.

Conclusion

People who have dementia can benefit hugely from rehabilitation. Rehabilitation is an integral part of the work of the nurse and is something that nurses are well placed to promote, even within the constraints of the acute hospital environment. However, the rehabilitation of people who have dementia raises some specific care issues which may need to be addressed through education and training of acute sector nurses. Knowledge of the literature about positive approaches to dementia may be lacking and understanding of lifespan and quality of life issues may be limited. Dementia raises some new challenges for nurses. The way in which nurses conceptualize dementia may be important in determining the nature of nurse–patient interaction and nurses may not have considered this during the pre-registration period. Ethical issues such as rationing of rehabilitation resources and the management of workload are also important challenges. While the acute hospital ward is not an ideal setting for the rehabilitation of people with dementia, nurses in these settings can spend some concentrated periods of time working with patients to achieve rehabilitation goals. Despite the acuity of the setting and the environmental problems raised by an acute hospital ward the need to rehabilitate patients in acute care areas is a reality in today's health service.

Nurses in acute hospital settings can assist with the rehabilitation of patients and work closely with members of the multidisciplinary team to facilitate effective discharge planning for people admitted to hospital. Rehabilitation is a definitive part of the role of nurses in a wide variety of care settings. Education in specific aspects of dementia and positive approaches to care could allow acute sector nurses the resources they need to unlock the considerable rehabilitation potential of people who live with dementia.

References

Asch, S.E. (1946) 'Basic concepts and approaches in social cognition: Forming impressions of personality.' In M. Hewstone, A.S.R. Manstead and W. Stroebe (eds) *The Blackwell Reader in Social Psychology*. Oxford: Blackwell Publishers.

Cohen, D. and Eisdorfer, C. (2002) *The Loss of Self*. New York: WW Norton & Co.

Diamond, P.T., Felsenthal, G., Macciocchi, S.N., Butler, D.H. and Lally-Cassady, D. (1996) 'Effect of cognitive impairment on rehabilitation outcome.' *American Journal of Physical and Medical Rehabilitation 75*, 40–43.

Goldstein, F.C., Strasser, D.C., Woodard, J.L. and Roberts, V.J. (1997) 'Functional outcome of cognitively impaired hip fracture patients on a geriatric rehabilitation unit.' *Journal of the American Geriatric Society 45*, 35–42.

Henderson, V. (1966) *The Nature of Nursing: A Definition and its Implications for Practice, Research and Education*. New York: Macmillan.

Livingston, C. (1991) 'Opportunities in rehabilitation nursing.' *American Journal of Nursing 91*, 2, 90, 92, 94–95.

Meyer, C. (1993) 'The changing face of rehabilitation nursing.' *American Journal of Nursing 93*, 2, 76–78, 80, 82.

Preston, K. (1994) 'Rehabilitation nursing – a client-centered philosophy.' *American Journal of Nursing 94*, 2, 66, 68–70.

Sabat, S.R. (1994) 'Excess disability and malignant social-psychology – A case-study of Alzheimers Disease.' *Journal of Community and Applied Social Psychology 4*, 3, 157–166.

Sabat, S.R. (1998) 'Voices of Alzheimer's disease sufferers: A call for treatment based on personhood.' *Journal of Clinical Ethics 9*, 1, 35–48.

Vittoria, A.K. (1999) '"Our own little language": Naming and the social construction of Alzheimer's disease.' *Symbolic Interaction 22*, 4, 361–384.

Watson, R. (1997) 'Is dementia a challenge to the identity of the mental health nurse.' In S. Tilley (ed) *The Mental Health Nurse: Views of Practice and Education*. Oxford: Blackwell Science.

Wood, L.A. and Ryan, E.B. (1991) 'Talk to elders: Social structures, attitudes and forms of address.' *Ageing and Society 11*, 167–187.

CHAPTER 21

The Role of Specialist Care Homes

Susan Nixon

Introduction

The aims and objectives of care planning within a specialist care home for people with dementia follow the basic theories of both social and physical rehabilitation. There are, however, different models of rehabilitation (Nolan, Nolan and Booth 1997) and this may be a factor in determining the reasons why the term is less used in dementia care. One definition suggests that the aim of rehabilitation is to restore effectiveness. This was originally the objective of long-term care of older people when the focus was to rehabilitate and send people home again. Specialist dementia care is concerned with working with the person in helping them to find methods of coping with the effects of dementia and to adapt to their new situation. It is also concerned with helping families and carers come to terms with the diagnosis of dementia.

Barriers to rehabilitation

In considering the reasons as to why rehabilitation is a term less used when discussing interventions with a person with dementia I am reminded of a situation where I was asked to reassess a lady with dementia who had had surgery to repair a break to her hip. On visiting her in hospital I found her in a chair, blocked in by an extremely heavy bed table. Unable to move the table, the lady was essentially being restrained. I asked to speak with the physiotherapist to ascertain what kind of rehabilitation she was receiving, and if she had a zimmer. The physiotherapist stated that she had not been given a zimmer as she had severe cognitive impairment and would forget to use it. Rehabilitation involved a short walk, once a day. Unfortunately the one thing that people with dementia need in any intervention is time, a great deal of time and often hospital staff are overworked and do not have the resources to provide that time. The lack of intensive rehabilitation could serve as a barrier and result in an older person remaining in hospital with very poor mobility.

A second consideration is the ambiguous definition of rehabilitation. Is it an intervention used to restore previous abilities or an intervention to help people adapt to new situations? Nolan (2001) highlights two paradigms of rehabilitation, the Restricted Isolated Model and the Comprehensive Integrative Model. The first model, he suggests, is the model that most services use whilst the second model is defined by literature as relating to the perceptions of patients and their carers. The Restricted Isolated Model suggests that intervention should be time limited and intervention should focus on the person's disability. In relation to people with dementia, where good practice is based on the concept of personhood, developed by Kitwood (1997), and should concentrate on abilities, this model would not be appropriate. The Comprehensive Integrative Model favoured by patients and their carers, in total contrast, suggests that any intervention should be long term and should consider the disability at an individual, community, environmental and societal level. It should also consider the views of family and carer. This would suggest that rehabilitation should be used to help people adapt to new situations.

Rehabilitation and dementia

There is very little written about rehabilitation and dementia; most literature relates to frail, older people. This could be due to the fact that there still exists the view, for some, that dementia is a degenerative disease with no cure, and therefore rehabilitation would be futile, as well as to the reasons stated above.

As a manager of a busy specialist care home I found it extremely difficult to apply a multidisciplinary approach. I often found that other professionals involved with clients when in the community were very quick to withdraw their expertise when the client was admitted to a care home. Waiting lists for their services and large caseloads prevented them from being able to offer continued support. In addition to this, professionals from both Health and Social Work would not prioritize a person once they were in residential care as they were seen as receiving a service already whilst others stayed on a waiting list.

Killeen (1996) lists rehabilitation as one integral aspect of multidisciplinary assessment and support, which seeks to empower the person with dementia. Joint working and effective communication are paramount to any work but particularly important when offering rehabilitative care. A recent visit to a care home in

Norway that used technology to support daily living applied this theory. Every-day activities involved the residents collectively making meals, baking cakes, cleaning and gardening. Care staff worked together with technicians, medics and families to empower the residents and to help them to live as independently as possible. As each person's needs changed the care plan changed after consultation with everyone involved. Rehabilitation was instinctive and people worked together offering continuity of care without question.

Rehabilitation within specialist care homes

There is no doubt that good care practice within a specialist care home takes the form of rehabilitation concerned with helping people adapt to the changes imposed on them by dementia. Kitwood (1997) suggests that there are two kinds of change that occur side by side. The first relates to the deterioration of memory, reasoning and comprehension and the second to patterns of relationship and interaction. The aims and objectives of any care planning should therefore reflect these changes and care workers should be involved not only with the person themselves, but also with their family and carers. The care worker must use skills in detection in order to place together the pieces of a very intricate puzzle when the person is first admitted to care. They must work alongside the family/carer and the care manager responsible for the initial assessment as well as any other professionals involved. Information gleaned at this point is paramount to the care plan and to understanding what kind of loss or change the person with dementia is experiencing. It may include: changes in their likes and dislikes; what tasks they are able to do for themselves irrespective of how minor some may be; what tasks they are now unable to do for themselves or could manage with help and support; people involved in their life and their role; social roles they may have had or continue to have; and places that are important to them. This list is by no means exhaustive but collectively helps to paint a full picture of the person as an individual, both before the onset of dementia and after.

It has been stated that a move into any communal setting involves some loss of autonomy (Wilson 2000). Care planning in relation to the person with demen-tia should strive to give a person back their autonomy and reflect the changes at each stage of the dementia. It should be person-centred and use a range of thera-peutic interventions which aim to enable people to regain old skills as well as maintain current ones. One aspect of the care offered in the Norwegian care home that greatly impressed me was the fact that each of the eight people living together had a role. The care offered gave each person the opportunity to make independent decisions in relation to tasks concerned with everyday living. One person was responsible for preparing the vegetables at lunch whilst three others were preparing fruit for the dessert, the more difficult tasks were undertaken by a volunteer staff member. They did not need constant reassurance or reminding, they knew their tasks and did them. The carers skilfully encouraged each person with the use of humour, and by real conversation regarding ordinary actions.

Carers should also be involved in any care planning, particularly if they have had a great deal of involvement in providing care prior to admission. Some care homes are reluctant to include carers in providing care due to a variety of reasons, including health and safety or risk assessment. Carers are often reluctant to offer help in case the care home staff see this as being intrusive. Encouraging carers to be included in continuing care offers consistency both in terms of care practice as well as for the person with dementia in any rehabilitative care.

Rehabilitation in day care and short breaks

There are other settings where rehabilitation is extremely important, and if offered could enable a person with dementia to continue either living independently with support or living with a carer for longer. Referral to day and short break care has been shown to extend the duration of people with dementia living independently (Levin, Sinclair and Gorbach 1992).

In a study of residents in a nursing home setting, who did not have dementia, it was found that a significant number of people with low level needs had been assessed as having greater needs (Penrice et al. 2001). Following admission they improved greatly, suggesting that perhaps with the correct rehabilitation they could have remained in their own home. The same could be said of people with dementia when assessments highlight risk factors. This assessed level of risk determines the decision about whether or not an application should be made for long-term care. Some practitioners and carers are willing to take more risks than others. In my experience, two of the most common reasons for people with dementia being admitted into long-term care are social isolation and wandering behaviour. Carers find the risks involved with wandering particularly difficult to cope with. A short period of respite or attendance in day care can sometimes help to determine the reasons for 'wandering', as well as incontinence, increased confusion or poor mobility.

Sometimes there is a tendency for care workers, when preparing care plans, to concentrate on physical rehabilitation. It is common for people with dementia to experience symptoms of anxiety and depression, especially in the early stages of the illness (McKeith and Fairbairn 2001). This can remain undetected for long periods as some of the normal features of ageing, such as poor sleep, apathy and tearfulness, can be similar (Hopker 1999). It is important that care plans also identify issues relating to social rehabilitation such as low self-esteem, isolation and signs of depressive behaviour. In addition, it is also possible that many people have been misdiagnosed as having dementia when they actually have a condition responsive to treatment for depression (Kitwood 1997). In such cases clues can be gathered from the pattern of daily living: people who are depressed tend to be low and confused in the morning, but improve towards the evening, whilst people with dementia tend to be at their best in the early part of the day.

The same principles of care planning in relation to long-term care and rehabilitation can be applied to short breaks and day care. People with dementia who live independently can often suffer from a degree of malnutrition, particularly when no one is monitoring their eating patterns. They may also experience difficulties in relation to polypharmacy where several different medications are working against each other. The over use of medication in people with dementia has been greatly documented, therefore any rehabilitation should include a review of the person's drug treatments. These issues are very common in relation to people with dementia, particularly those who live independently. The short break and day care can therefore be used as a period of physical rehabilitation.

This process will only be effective if the care plan is then passed to the carer to continue, otherwise the same problems will recur, and the person with dementia will not benefit from the short break or day care service.

Conclusions

Within a specialist care home environment, rehabilitation for people with dementia is paramount to person-centred care and should adopt a multidisciplinary approach. For rehabilitation to be effective care workers need to be proficient in devising care plans which take into account physical, social and emotional needs. It should be a continual process with care plans concentrating on the person's abilities, maintaining autonomy and changing as the person with dementia changes. Involving other professionals and carers is an integral part of any rehabilitation process, particularly in relation to helping people with dementia adapt to the changes in their life.

References

Hopker, S. (1999) *Drug Treatments and Dementia*. London: Jessica Kingsley Publishers.

Killeen, J. (1996) 'Involving people with dementia and their carers in developing services.' In C. Cantley (ed) *A Handbook of Dementia Care*. Buckingham: Open University Press.

Kitwood, T. (1997) *Dementia Reconsidered: The Person Comes First*. Buckingham: Open University Press.

Levin, E., Sinclair, I. and Gorbach, P. (1992) *Better for the Break*. London: HMSO.

McKeith, I. and Fairbairn, A. (2001) 'Biomedical and clinical perspectives.' In C. Cantley (ed) *A Handbook of Dementia Care*. Buckingham: Open University Press.

Nolan, M. (2001) 'Acute and rehabilitative care of older people.' In M. Nolan, S. Davies and G. Grant (eds) *Working with Older People and their Families: Key Issues in Policy and Practice*. Buckingham: Open University Press.

Nolan, M.R., Nolan, J. and Booth, A. (1997) 'Preparation for multi-professional/multi agency health care practice: the nursing contribution to rehabilitation within the multidisciplinary team, literature review and curriculum analysis. Final report to the English National Board.' In M. Nolan, S. Davies and G. Grant (eds) *Working with Older People and their Families: Key Issues in Policy and Practice*. Buckingham: Open University Press.

Penrice, G.M., Simpson, L., de Caestecker, L., Brown, G. and Gillies, S. (2001) 'Low dependency residents in private nursing homes in Glasgow.' *Health Bulletin 59*, 1, 4–9.

Wilson, G. (2000) *Understanding Old Age: Critical and Global Perspectives*. London: Sage Publications.

PART FIVE

Specific Interventions

CHAPTER 22

Fit for Life: The Contribution of Life Story Work

Faith Gibson

In considering a rehabilitative approach to people who develop dementia it is important to know about the time of their lives before dementia developed – the long and complex journeys travelled to reach the present. Such knowledge can be used to influence the quality of here and now experience, to reinforce a sense of identity and to help structure a programme of occupation, relevant activities and acceptable recreation that helps to preserve and enhance well-being. Additionally, mutual engagement in life story work involving family members of various ages and circumstances and professional carers can assist in delaying the erosion of relationships and encroaching isolation that so frequently accompanies the onset of dementia, whether this occurs in late life or mid life and whatever its nature and accompanying complications.

If rehabilitation is defined as the process of restoring someone to health or normal life, it seems hardly credible that this is possible in the face of a condition such as dementia, usually thought to be irreversible and terminal. To delay rather than prevent the advance of dementia perhaps is the most that can be hoped for. If someone, however, can be helped to retain, or even regain a sense of happiness and security that easily evaporates with the onset of dementia, this can be a worthwhile achievement to which life story work can contribute. How others treat people with dementia and the surroundings in which they live cause many problems additional to basic cognitive loss (Sabat 2001). People may lose confidence, develop anxiety and fail to be appreciated as unique individuals. Having and using a detailed knowledge of earlier patterns of relating and responding in ways informed by a person's life history can prevent many of these additional or secondary complications.

Life story work is a loose phrase that refers to various ways of engaging and interacting with people of different ages in order to encourage and assist them to recall and to record in tangible form their personal histories. The deliberately planned process may be as short or long, simple or sophisticated as suits the person and the present circumstances. Individuals are encouraged to look back, to talk about their memories and to preserve these recollections in words or images so as to have an aide memoire to remind themselves and others of the past and to encourage further recall and reflection.

The person with dementia is central to this process although others such as family or professional carers can also derive considerable benefit from being involved. The process and its tangible outcomes assist communication and aid the development of positive relationships. Life story work therefore has multiple benefits for various people. It is an activity that, although largely about the past, takes place in the present. It involves a series of intensive, non-threatening, highly personal discussions between the person disabled by dementia and a responsive, appreciative listener. The primary purpose of these sociable meetings is to listen attentively, validate the story being recounted and assist with its preservation in an attractive, accessible, acceptable format.

Life story books were originally developed as a tool for working with children whose sense of identity, family relationships and emotional security had been fractured by problematic life events and adults' inability consistently to nurture and care. This approach is now used with people of all ages. A book or more frequently a loose-leaf binder with plastic pockets is used to organize and preserve the material collected, but other formats and newer technologies including audiotape, video film, multimedia archiving programmes and CD-ROMS are sometimes used.

People are encouraged to reminisce about their lives, to collect, discuss and annotate, as far as possible in their own words, photographic and documentary material. The record, in whatever format, needs to represent the broad life experience of its owner. It is usually arranged chronologically from childhood to the present, or sometimes themes such as family life, significant people, important places, work and recreation are used. The person is encouraged to recount the story of his or her life and in the process to re-evaluate it to some extent. Showing actual photographs and memorabilia usually prompts and accelerates the recall process. If no personal memory triggers are available, then pictures and memorabilia of related or similar experience can be used to prompt recall. The story is then reproduced in the words of the person and photographs, letters and documents are incorporated in the record to illustrate, illuminate and enliven the text (Murphy and Moyes 1997).

In a number of regular weekly sessions (at least six are recommended), information is gathered, discussed and organized. The record becomes an organic dynamic account that can have further material added at any future time. A comprehensive life story needs to include information about:

- childhood, parents and siblings
- adolescence
- young adulthood, relationships, family life and children
- middle age
- later years
- ethnicity, religion, special skills, interests and achievements.

People with dementia usually need considerable assistance in executing the writing of their story so the willing listener usually doubles as an amanuensis. This is not an easy role to fulfil. It must be founded on a trusting relationship that grows and develops out of working together. Careful listening, respect and willingness to serve as an enabler or facilitator are essential. Depending on the wishes, needs and present living arrangements of the person with dementia, the helper may need to be very active in seeking out relevant material and in prompting discussion.

Trips and pilgrimages to past places of significance may be an important way of gathering information, both past and present. Family members and old friends may need to be enlisted as aides and sources of information. The actual representation and arrangement of the material requires sensitive discussion with the person whose life story is being recounted. Above all the helper must be willing and able to hear the stories that the person wants to tell, no matter what the content, nor how painful the process may become in terms of reviving memories of past pain and unresolved difficulties (Gibson 2003).

It is this risk of precipitating sadness or depression that initially deters some professional carers from embarking on life story work. They fear that they will not be able to handle the emotions aroused or that the person will be unable to resolve the painful memories and be left permanently upset. There is some small risk involved but this is far outweighed by the positive benefits that ordinarily accrue. During such work it is good practice to have access to a supervisor or mentor who can offer support and guidance during the process of sharing and bearing another person's pain. On the very rare occasions when serious emotional disturbance is triggered in either the teller or the hearer, recourse to a skilled clinical professional should be available.

There is a great temptation for workers to get caught up in the production of the 'record' or product, no matter what form it takes. The process of engagement may be eclipsed in the enthusiasm to produce an impressive, comprehensive, attractive product. While the process must always be more important than the product, the significance of the record and its possible longer-term benefits for the person, carers and family members should not be underestimated. The quality of the present encounter, week by week, can be enhanced by shared involvement in a task of personal significance in which conversation is set within familiar territory and the person with dementia is revealed in all his or her unique individuality and rich varied life experience. Highly sensitive information may need to be excluded from the record but not from the discussion. Because of failing or freakish memory, the tangible record can serve as a memory jogger, a focus for initiating future conversation and as proof of a life lived, problems overcome, experience validated and achievements recognized.

At the heart of high quality dementia care lies recognition of the need to arrange care in ways which encourage people to continue to do 'ordinary' things. Only very late into the condition, unless extreme physical frailty also exists, should people be denied opportunities to continue to do whatever interests them and gives them pleasure. The range of such possible activities, occupations and recreation will probably be more diverse in younger people but the type of constructive occupation chosen is more likely to arise from lifelong personality and lifetime preferences rather than being determined by chronological age alone.

Thus the physical capacity of younger people with dementia usually requires more extensive provision of suitable physical activity and exercise while also recognising the acute anxiety, apprehension and possible depression that may accompany a recent diagnosis. For example, the younger person who has always led a sedentary life is more likely to continue to wish to do so. The golfer, fisherman or active housewife may retain an interest in these earlier activities, despite developing dementia. Each may welcome the opportunity to continue earlier pursuits if only carers have sufficient imagination to make this possible. Life story work can provide illuminating information and satisfying involvement regardless of age, stage or type of dementia.

The role of friends and families in life story work remains largely an under-exploited resource in dementia care. These people are an obvious source of information but they are also likely to be beneficiaries if they too can share in the process. The negative effects of dementia upon family carers are well documented (Bruce 1997). They frequently report prolonged grief for changing or lost relationships, increasing social isolation, feelings of subjective burden, stress and exhaustion. Accounts of acceptance of change and satisfaction from caring are less common but not unknown. Shared life story work can assist carers to hold onto and celebrate good times past (providing the relationship has been predominantly satisfactory). It may also assist them to understand the reasons for past dissatisfactions, help them to rehabilitate or restore fractured relationships and accept inevitable changes.

Family members may also benefit if they too can be involved in the life story process. Whether these family members are adult children or younger grandchildren, they may gain invaluable information about their family history. They may find an intriguing way of actually spending time with their ageing, deteriorating relative. They may discover that dementia is less frightening or threatening and they may begin to accept their own inescapable ageing and mortality. The record too may become an important reminder of their antecedents and their connections across the generations.

In care contexts there are many ways of using a life story. Bell and Troxel (1996, 2001) suggest the following:

- greeting the person and improving recognition
- introducing the person to others (especially in day services and residential contexts)
- reminiscing
- improving communication through clues and cues
- designing appropriate activities
- pointing out past accomplishments
- helping to prevent challenging behaviours
- incorporating past daily rituals
- broadening the caregiving network and resources.

To summarize, life story work builds appreciation, acknowledges unique individuality and assists failing memory by providing a tangible record of the past. It builds links between the past and the present. This is achieved primarily by utilizing long-term memory to communicate in the present. Life story work places the person with dementia at the centre of the story told and, through the process of developing a loving respectful relationship, it achieves a useful tangible working tool that benefits the person with dementia, and their family and professional carers.

References

Bell, V. and Troxel, D. (1996) *The Best Friends Approach to Alzheimer's Care.* Baltimore: Health Professions Press.

Bell, V. and Troxel, D. (2001) *The Best Friends Staff: Building a Culture of Care in Alzheimer's Programs.* Baltimore: Health Professions Press.

Bruce, E. (1997) 'Reminiscence and family carers.' In P. Schweitzer (ed) *Reminiscence in Dementia Care.* London: Age Exchange, 50–57.

Gibson, F. (2004) *Reminiscence in Health, Social Care and Community Contexts.* Baltimore: Health Professions Press.

Murphy, C.J. and Moyes, M. (1997) 'Life story work.' In M. Marshall (ed) *State of the Art in Dementia Care.* London: CPA.

Sabat, S.R. (2001) 'Surviving manifestations of selfhood in Alzheimer's disease.' *Dementia 1,* 1, 25–36.

CHAPTER 23

Cognitive Rehabilitation for People with Dementia

Linda Clare

Rehabilitation is about 'enabling people who are disabled by injury or disease to achieve their optimum physical, psychological, social and vocational well-being' (McLellan 1991). This concept can be applied to people at different life stages and with different types of problems or disorders. It is very relevant for older people with dementia. In fact, Cohen and Eisdorfer (1986) argued that rehabilitation was the most appropriate framework within which to think about dementia care.

Rehabilitation can focus on a range of different areas of need, and goals can be adjusted flexibly in response to changing needs. Recently, researchers have started to describe the application of cognitive rehabilitation for people with dementia, especially in the early stages where changes in memory and cognitive functioning have a prominent impact on well-being. This is based on the under-standing that despite difficulties with memory and other cognitive functions, people with dementia still have the ability to learn new associations and informa-tion, and to adjust their behaviour and responses.

Cognitive rehabilitation aims to 'enable clients or patients, and their families, to live with, manage, by-pass, reduce or come to terms with deficits precipitated by injury to the brain' (Wilson 1997). This definition was written to describe work with people who had experienced a brain injury, but it is also relevant to people who develop dementia. In this context, cognitive rehabilitation is essen-tially about using our understanding of cognitive functioning to support people in the process of living with dementia. This focus on 'living with' dementia points to the relevance of viewing dementia in terms of disability.

A biopsychosocial model of disability (World Health Organization 1980, 1998) makes the important distinction between underlying impairment at the neurological or physical level, activity (disability) and participation (handicap). Activity and participation are influenced by the personal and social context and do not follow directly or straightforwardly from impairment. Negative contexts can contribute to producing unnecessary excess disability (Reifler and Larson 1990). This of course is also a central tenet of Kitwood's dialectical model of dementia, which emphasizes the interplay between neurological impairment on the one hand and social psychology on the other (Kitwood 1997).

Cognitive rehabilitation for people with dementia is not typically aiming to cure or reduce impairment at the neurological level. Rather, the aim is to work together to find ways of dealing with the problems that arise as a result of cognitive changes, so as to enable the person to participate in interactions and engage in desired activities as best they can, within their own personal and social context. This means that cognitive rehabilitation needs to include a focus on emotional responses, such as loss, anger, frustration or anxiety, and to take into account the impact on the person's family or wider system, as well as identifying specific strategies for dealing with difficulties resulting from changes in memory or other cognitive domains.

Person-centred approaches in dementia care highlight the importance of individual identity and selfhood. One important aim of cognitive rehabilitation is to empower individuals by strengthening the sense of self and identity and enhancing feelings of being in control. Therefore, cognitive rehabilitation needs to be undertaken in a way that is sensitive to, and supportive of, individual coping, so it is important to start with an understanding of how people with early-stage dementia may attempt to adjust and cope with what is happening to them.

We can think of coping responses in early-stage dementia as being on a continuum (Clare 2002, 2003; Pearce, Clare and Pistrang 2002). At one end are 'self-maintaining' strategies aimed at keeping things the same as before and holding onto a past sense of self. At the other are 'self-adjusting' strategies aimed at trying to face head on the changes that are occurring and integrate these into a developing sense of self. Individuals use a range of coping strategies that may be placed at different points along this continuum, and may draw on different strategies at different times and in different situations. Most, though, will show a preference for more maintaining or more adjusting strategies. Cognitive rehabilitation interventions can be designed to support either type of coping, and should always aim to be consistent with an individual's preferred coping style.

A key strength of the cognitive rehabilitation approach is that interventions are individually tailored and focus directly on real, everyday situations and difficulties in a collaborative manner. The starting point involves identifying desired outcomes. This means that interventions focus on things that are causing concern to the person with dementia and his or her family members, and goals are relevant to improving quality of life. Specific interventions are then devised, based on an understanding of a profile of cognitive functioning that indicates both strengths and difficulties, and taking into account the person's preferred coping styles, other psychological and emotional needs, and support system. In this context, it is important to note that a specific diagnosis, as such, is not an essential prerequisite for cognitive rehabilitation, although it may provide some helpful guidance; what is more important is a formulation of the cognitive difficulties in relation to other psychological and social factors. Some acknowledgement of difficulties is, however, important. People cope in different ways, and if an individual is coping by maintaining that there are no significant changes in functioning and no problem areas, cognitive rehabilitation is probably not going to be the right approach at that time. In this kind of situation, it may be more useful to offer advice and support to family members, while remaining in contact with the person with dementia so as to build a relationship and be ready to offer support when coping strategies shift. In our research, we found that a higher level of explicit awareness of memory difficulties was related to better outcome in a cognitive rehabilitation intervention (Clare *et al.* 2004).

Cognitive rehabilitation interventions draw on a range of principles, methods and techniques, all with demonstrated efficacy for people with dementia, such as spaced retrieval (Camp 1989; Camp, Bird and Cherry 2000), to create a plan for tackling the agreed goals. This is likely to involve either making the most of remaining cognitive skills, identifying compensatory strategies or altering the environment so as to better support cognitive functioning. Throughout this process, there is scope for discussion of emotional responses, and specific attention can be paid to particular issues that are impacting on the intervention or on the person's general functioning, such as high levels of anxiety or embarrassment in social situations. Of course, this also offers an opportunity to build a good working relationship that provides the foundation for supporting the person and family over time as the dementia progresses. I will illustrate this process with an example from our research (Clare *et al.* 2000) that shows how what was essentially a very simple intervention could make a significant difference to everyday life.

Evelyn had a diagnosis of early-stage Alzheimer's disease and a number of physical health problems. She kept up with an extensive range of interests, but was very bothered by the effects of her memory difficulties. When I first met her, she was acutely aware that she repeatedly asked her husband, Ed, the same question over and over again, usually 'What day is it today?' She said that she thought this must be 'soul destroying' for him, and she desperately wanted to stop doing it, but could not help herself asking, and she did genuinely want to know what day it was each time she asked. Ed was very frustrated by Evelyn's questioning, and although he tried to remain patient, he was finding this increasingly hard.

Evelyn was coping with the onset of dementia by facing up to its impact and trying to adapt, and her cognitive profile, despite severe difficulties in memory, showed numerous important strengths, including the capacity for some new learning, good organizational skills and intact visuospatial perception. This suggested that she should be able to learn and make use of a strategy that could take the place of her repetitive questioning. The strategy we decided on was to introduce a calendar that Evelyn could consult whenever she wanted to know what day it was, allowing her to find out the information independently. A central part of the intervention involved getting Evelyn into the habit of using her calendar. It was positioned in a prominent place, and Ed agreed to prompt Evelyn three times each day to look at her calendar and find out what day it was. In addition, if Evelyn asked at other times, Ed was to suggest that she look at her calendar. The intervention therefore combined a regular schedule of prompting, an errorless learning paradigm whereby Evelyn would be directed to the calendar every time she wanted to know the day, and the intrinsic reinforcement provided by using the calendar to get the desired information. This continued for three weeks, at the end of which Evelyn was using the calendar regularly and was able to explain what she needed to do in order to find out what day it was. This meant that now, when she wanted to find out the day, she was able to reject the idea of asking Ed and instead direct herself to look at her calendar. In order to make sure this was maintained, Ed's regular prompting was faded out gradually over a number of weeks, until eventually Evelyn was continuing to use the calendar entirely by herself. This made Evelyn feel more in control, and Ed commented that things were '100 per cent better'. The idea that a solution could be found for some of their practical difficulties led Evelyn and Ed to raise other concerns related to the impact of Evelyn's memory problems, and we engaged together in a problem-solving process to try to come up with strategies for dealing with them. Over time, they began to do this more and more by themselves, and although Evelyn's memory difficulties remained, their daily life became a little easier and less stressful, and they were both able to carry on doing the things they enjoyed.

We have also applied this kind of approach to help people with early-stage dementia to learn or re-learn information that is important to them. For example, some have chosen to learn names of people they meet regularly as a way of helping to maintain social involvement (Clare et al. 1999, Clare et al. 2001, Clare et al. 2003a). Other participants have chosen to focus on family-related information so as to better engage in conversation, or have identified practical goals such as being able to recognize and differentiate coins in order to manage their shopping better. Activities of daily living have been targeted by Josephsson et al. (1993). 'Problem' behaviours arising as a result of cognitive difficulties can also be targeted in a similar way (Bird 2001). This approach is not restricted to people with early-stage dementia, but is equally relevant for people with more advanced dementia (Bird 2000). One example here is the use of memory books as a means of stimulating conversation between people with dementia and their caregivers, thus contributing to a reduction in excess disability in residential care settings (Bourgeois 1990, 1991, 1992).

The limited evidence that is currently available, mainly drawn from reports of single case experimental designs, suggests that cognitive rehabilitation interventions can produce significant improvements in targeted areas, at least for a proportion of participants. Clearly there is a great deal more work to be done here, but recent reviews are positive about the potential for cognitive rehabilitation (De Vreese *et al.* 2001). This contrasts with the finding that cognitive training interventions do not provide any significant benefits for people with mild to moderate dementia (Clare *et al.* 2003b). Cognition-focused interventions for people with mild to moderate dementia have hitherto typically adopted a cognitive training rather than a cognitive rehabilitation model, involving practice on standardized tasks and exercises relating to various domains of cognitive functioning. The cognitive training approach has a number of important limitations, as it allows little scope for adjusting to individual needs or coping styles, nor does it address emotional responses in an integrated way. In addition, it cannot be assumed that any gains that might result from training would generalize to everyday situations or have any clinically significant impact. The currently available evidence suggests that the way forward lies not in cognitive training but in a more individualized, cognitive rehabilitation approach.

The evidence that we do have for cognitive rehabilitation clearly shows that we are justified in believing that something can be done. Cognitive rehabilitation will not remove memory and cognitive problems, but it can make a considerable difference to quality of life and help people maintain involvement and well-being. The value of rehabilitation for people with dementia has recently been eloquently expressed by Morris Friedell, who has a diagnosis of Alzheimer's disease and is a director of Dementia Advocacy and Support Network International. He writes:

> I have come to believe that rehabilitation can have a powerful effect on a patient's quality of life, allowing him or her to regain much lost ground and then maintain for years. What is needed is not some expensive institute, but some concepts which are not too complicated, the support of a good friend or psychotherapist, and lots of hope and hard work.

In applying cognitive rehabilitation, we already have at our disposal a number of concepts and methods that are not too complicated, along with a developing understanding of how best to support people with dementia. This offers a strong incentive for further developing the potential of cognitive rehabilitation as a means of helping people who are living with dementia.

References

Bird, M. (2001) 'Behavioural difficulties and cued recall of adaptive behaviour in dementia: experimental and clinical evidence.' *Neuropsychological Rehabilitation 11*, 357–375.

Bird, M.J. (2000) 'Psychosocial rehabilitation for problems arising from cognitive deficits in dementia.' In R.D. Hill, L. Bäckman and A.S. Neely (eds) *Cognitive Rehabilitation in Old Age*. Oxford: Oxford University Press.

Bourgeois, M.S. (1990) 'Enhancing conversation skills in patients with Alzheimer's disease using a prosthetic memory aid.' *Journal of Applied Behavior Analysis 23*, 29–42.

Bourgeois, M.S. (1991) 'Communication treatment for adults with dementia.' *Journal of Speech and Hearing Research 34*, 831–844.

Bourgeois, M.S. (1992) 'Evaluating memory wallets in conversations with persons with dementia.' *Journal of Speech and Hearing Research 35*, 1344–1357.

Camp, C.J. (1989) 'Facilitation of new learning in Alzheimer's disease.' In G. Gilmore, P. Whitehouse and M. Wykle (eds) *Memory and Aging: Theory, Research and Practice*. New York: Springer.

Camp, C.J., Bird, M.J. and Cherry, K.E. (2000) 'Retrieval strategies as a rehabilitation aid for cognitive loss in pathological aging.' In R.D. Hill, L. Bäckman and A.S. Neely (eds) *Cognitive Rehabilitation in Old Age*. Oxford: Oxford University Press.

Clare, L. (2002) 'We'll fight it as long as we can: Coping with the onset of Alzheimer's disease.' *Aging and Mental Health 6*, 139–148.

Clare, L. (2003) 'Managing threats to self: Awareness in early-stage Alzheimer's disease.' *Social Science and Medicine 57*, 1017–1029.

Clare, L., Wilson, B.A., Breen, K. and Hodges, J.R. (1999) 'Errorless learning of face-name associations in early Alzheimer's disease.' *Neurocase 5*, 37–46.

Clare, L., Wilson, B.A., Carter, G., Gosses, A., Breen, K. and Hodges, J.R. (2000) 'Intervening with everyday memory problems in early Alzheimer's disease: An errorless learning approach.' *Journal of Clinical and Experimental Neuropsychology 22*, 132–146.

Clare, L., Wilson, B.A., Carter, G. and Hodges, J.R. (2003a) 'Cognitive rehabilitation as a component of early intervention in dementia: A single case study.' *Aging and Mental Health 7*, 15–21.

Clare, L., Wilson, B.A., Carter, G., Hodges, J.R. and Adams, M. (2001) 'Long-term maintenance of treatment gains following a cognitive rehabilitation intervention in early dementia of Alzheimer type: A single case study.' *Neuropsychological Rehabilitation 11*, 477–494.

Clare, L., Wilson, B.A., Carter, G., Roth, I. and Hodges, J.R. (2004) 'Awareness in early-stage Alzheimer's disease: Relationship to outcome of cognitive rehabilitation.' *Journal of Clinical and Experimental Neuropsychology 26*, 215–226.

Clare, L., Woods, R.T., Moniz-Cook, E.D., Orrell, M. and Spector, A. (2003b) 'Cognitive rehabilitation and cognitive training for early-stage Alzheimer's disease and vascular dementia' (Cochrane review). *Cochrane Library*, Issue 4. Chichester: Wiley.

Cohen, D. and Eisdorfer, C. (1986) *The Loss of Self: A Family Resource for the Care of Alzheimer's Disease and Related Disorders*. New York: W.W. Norton & Co.

De Vreese, L.P., Neri, M., Fioravanti, M., Belloi, L. and Zanetti, O. (2001) 'Memory rehabilitation in Alzheimer's disease: A review of progress.' *International Journal of Geriatric Psychiatry 16*, 794–809.

Josephsson, S., Bäckman, L., Borell, L., Bernspang, B., Nygard, L. and Ronnberg, L. (1993) 'Supporting everyday activities in dementia: an intervention study.' *International Journal of Geriatric Psychiatry 8*, 395–400.

Kitwood, T. (1997) *Dementia Reconsidered: The Person Comes First.* Buckingham: Open University Press.

McLellan, D.L. (1991) 'Functional recovery and the principles of disability medicine.' In M. Swash and J. Oxbury (eds) *Clinical Neurology 1*, London: Churchill Livingstone.

Pearce, A., Clare, L. and Pistrang, N. (2002) 'Managing sense of self: Coping in the early stages of Alzheimer's disease.' *Dementia 1*, 173–192.

Reifler, B.V. and Larson, E. (1990) 'Excess disability in dementia of the Alzheimer's type.' In E. Light and B.D. Lebowitz (eds) *Alzheimer's Disease Treatment and Family Stress.* New York: Hemisphere.

Wilson, B.A. (1997) 'Cognitive rehabilitation: How it is and how it might be.' *Journal of the International Neuropsychological Society 3*, 487–496.

World Health Organization (1980) *International Classification of Impairments, Disabilities, and Handicaps.* Geneva: World Health Organization.

World Health Organization (1998) *International Classification of Impairments, Disabilities and Handicaps* (2nd edn). Geneva: World Health Organization.

CHAPTER 24

Rehabilitation: Environmental Aids and Adaptations

Mary Marshall

In the same way that people with mobility problems are offered a handrail, people with dementia may need a more prosthetic environment in relation to their dementia. As with other kinds of disability, this may take the form of removing items which can exacerbate the disability as well as modifying the environment to compensate for it. The aim is always to assist the person to function as independently as possible.

Background

People with dementia may be functioning less than optimally because of their environment after an acute episode related to their dementia or some physical problem, or because nobody has addressed the environmental issues. There are many disabilities that result from dementia, for which the environment can compensate. The most common disabilities are:

- impaired memory/recall
- impaired learning
- impaired reasoning
- increasing dependence on the senses
- high levels of stress.

The use of the word 'impaired' is deliberate because of one of the themes of this book is that people with dementia have remaining competence which needs to be recognized and maximized.

Some aids and adaptations

The environment can compensate in many ways. If someone has an impaired memory, they need to be able to see where they want to go and what they need rather than depending on their memory. It can be helpful to remove cupboard doors or install glass doors. This can be especially useful in those kitchens where all the appliances are hidden behind identical doors. People with dementia may need a very obvious hook for the front door keys. Losing things is a very stressful part of dementia and technologies can help, such as a locator devices for spectacles or purses (Knott 2003).

If you have to depend on seeing things to remember them or to find your way, lots of light is obviously important. People with dementia manage a great deal better when there is good lighting (Netten 1993). It can also be helpful to have some features highlighted for you. Light switches that are a contrasting colour to the wall or have a coloured band around them can be helpful.

If someone has impaired learning they should not have to learn where things are and they may find signs helpful. The most important place that they may need help to find is the toilet. The clearest signs are black on yellow, with the word toilet written with a capital and lower case to follow. Some people can no longer read, so a picture of a toilet may be helpful. Some people can manage neither so a landmark may be needed such as a plant or piece of furniture. These people may need coaching to remember the cue. Some people with dementia cannot find the toilet when they wake up in the night. They need to see it. Ideally a toilet should be visible from the bed. It should also be very clearly a toilet so it should contrast with the floor and wall and the seat and lid should be particularly clear.

If someone has impaired reasoning they may no longer be able to work out how to work a modern tap, especially if both hot and cold as well as volume are on the one stalk. They may no longer be able to work a modern light switch or shower control. It is, of course, not always possible to change fixtures and fittings, so simple explanatory signs may be needed.

Some people with dementia may no longer be able to work out the difference between rooms which they need to enter and those not available to them (cupboards, staff rooms). Rooms and cupboards that they do not need to enter can be a painted the same colour as the walls, so they are much less visible. Rooms that are important can be made obvious and perhaps signed as well. If replacing doors, glass panels can help so people can look through them and see what room lies behind. Frosted glass was always on the bathroom door in the past so this can be a useful cue for some people. There is often a problem of the fire door and this may need individualized attention for those who are drawn towards it. Some will not recognize it as a door if it is painted to look like a window, others may be deterred by a change of floor colour and texture, others may avoid it if it has a mirror on it and so on.

Some people with dementia struggle to work out time and are not helped by some of the clocks available. Luminous clocks may not be visible to sight impaired people. Some clock faces are too small. Other clocks are digital, which may not make sense. It may be an issue of night and day that is the problem and no clock is available which is both analogue and tells you whether it is am or pm. Some may need a low light by a big clock. People who can manage a digital clock can find the clock which shines the time on the ceiling very helpful. Some people find a chiming clock helpful. Other cues can be needed. Some people may need thicker curtains to keep out streetlight or early morning light. Others may need lights that are operated by a timer to go on in the morning.

People who are highly stressed can be hugely helped by a reduction in noise. This can be achieved by increasing the amount of fabric in the room as well as concealing the TV and radio so they are only used with care. In some establishments it may be possible to use sound absorbing panels in the ceiling and in partitions. They may also need quiet places to escape to such as a quiet lounge or the garden. Excessive and disabling noise is often the result of too many people in one place. Dining rooms are the worst offenders. Some dining rooms in care homes and hospitals cater for thirty people at once. Few people with dementia can remain calm and concentrate on their food with this amount of stimulation around them. Dining rooms should be as small as possible, and as quiet as possible. Eight seems to me to be a maximum and even then one or two people may need a separate space to eat because they are so distracted and disabled by others.

Stress can be reduced if people feel, in some way, in control of their environment. Window catches may need to be made easier so they can open the window if they need to. Doors which are safe to open like the one to the garden should be easy to open. Stress can also be induced if people feel confined. Every effort should be made to make aspects that reinforce confinement as hidden as possible. In care homes the front door can be out of sight, the garden fence concealed with planting and the fire doors set on the side rather than the end of corridors. These solutions are, of course, only possible if designing from scratch but imaginative care staff can find ways of adapting their environment to draw attention away from the obvious aspects which confine residents and patients.

Familiar personal objects which reinforce identity can be very helpful to calm someone who is highly stressed, possibly after several moves. Sometimes things to touch can be helpful such as a suitcase full of different scarves: velvet, silk, corduroy, tweed, knitted and so on.

Almost any disability results in increasing dependence on the senses, especially a cognitive disability. Awareness of this can lead to some imaginative approaches. If it is not known which sense is still functioning well it may be necessary to stimulate as many as possible. Thus someone who can no longer recall how and when to eat, can be much helped by stimulation of all the senses: touch by laying the table; sight by watching food being prepared or seeing a well laid table; smell by smell of food (ideally being prepared and always in the serving of it); hearing by the clink of cups, glasses, cutlery; taste perhaps by offering a sherry from a drinks trolley and kinaesthetic stimulation by actually doing things like stirring, or helping. All of these have implications for the environment which can be modified to make this approach to mealtimes possible.

Environments can be altered to provide all sorts of sensory stimulation. The most obvious is the bathroom. Here there are lots of opportunities if the room itself is pleasant and welcoming rather than intimidating. If there is an opportunity to refit the bathroom, attention needs to be given to the tiles which need to be attractive without being so 'busy' that they distract from important features such as the handrails. A bathroom needs to smell nice, which may require high shelves (in case the person eats the items) with pleasant smelling soap and bath oils. Some people are used to bathrooms full of seashells and other seaside memorabilia, and these can stimulate a lot of conversations. Some people like soothing music in the bathroom. On the other hand some people are highly stressed by the sound of running water so individualizing the stimulation is always essential. Gardens are another area which can provide multi-sensory stimulation in the form of plants that smell, jobs to do, textures to stroke, herbs to taste, the sound of wind bells or water features and lovely colours to look at.

Some care homes provide multi-sensory stimulation in the form of areas of the home with special features: an alcove that is set up like the seaside, a woodworking area smelling of sawdust and resin with lots of familiar tools and so on. Snoezelen rooms are not, in my experience, used a great deal. They have however alerted us all to the need to provide multi-sensory stimulation.

What is needed

Understanding how to compensate for disabilities always requires empathy and understanding of the experience of the disability itself. A checklist or list of suggestions is no substitute for standing in the shoes of someone with dementia and looking at the environment. It very quickly becomes clear that a lot of environments do not help people to find their way. Doors are all the same colour, toilets are out of sight, noise levels are overwhelming, sensory stimulation is absent and so on. Carers and staff can come up with wonderful and highly individualized solutions if they are alerted to the basic thinking.

Cognitive impairments are more difficult to simulate than other disabilities. People can get a glimmer of understanding of the world of someone in a wheelchair if they try it, as they can of the world of hearing impairment if they wear earplugs during the day. However we are all cognitively impaired from time to time: when we are excessively tired or stressed for example. We need to learn from these experiences to see what environmental factors helped us to cope. We have all struggled to find a toilet when anxious and in a new building, or our room in a hotel or bed and breakfast. We need to remember that for many people with dementia the place they now live may always feel like a new building. They may be unable to recall why they are there or where it is. Landmarks are more helpful than colour. We will recall our room in the bed and breakfast because it is beside a picture; we find our hotel room in relation to the lift or the fire extinguisher. The same approach helps people with dementia.

Conclusion

There are a great many things we can do to help people with dementia to be more independent in their environment. We need to know what their particular disabilities are so that we can use aid and adaptations to maximum effect. Often quite small things can make a big difference. We all know from experience that some buildings can disable anyone, so it is really a matter of learning from this to better appreciate what it must be like for someone with dementia. This realization can lead to countless imaginative solutions, a few of which have been mentioned in this chapter.

References

Knott, M. (2003) 'Smart as houses.' *EPSRC (Engineering and Physical Sciences Research Council) Newsline 28*, 22–23.

Netten, A. (1993) *A Positive Environment.* Aldershot: Ashgate Publishing.

CHAPTER 25

The Role of Medication in the Rehabilitation of People with Dementia

Cesar Rodriguez

Introduction

Rehabilitation of the older person with psychiatric disorder means restoring and maintaining the highest possible level of psychological, physical and social function despite the disabling effects of illness (Jones 2002). As with any other chronic and progressive condition, rehabilitation in dementia has to be flexible and change as necessary as the illness progresses. I believe rehabilitation should start as soon as someone is diagnosed with dementia. The particular roles of the doctor are to minimize potential side effects of drugs, treat physical and psychiatric conditions that interfere with rehabilitation, and use specific drugs known to improve cognition, behaviour and functioning in some people with dementia. Therefore, in this chapter I am going to discuss general aspects of medication in older people, especially those with dementia; the use of specific pharmacological treatments for psychological and behavioural symptoms of dementia; and, finally, the licensed medication for the symptomatic treatment of Alzheimer's disease.

Rehabilitation in dementia requires a multidisciplinary approach and that is well reflected in this book. The particular contributions that different profession-als bring to the field of rehabilitation in dementia should complement each other and, with a person-centred perspective, aim for the same outcome: maximizing the person's potential and minimizing disability.

Medication in older people: Special considerations

It is important not to assume that every physical or mental problem a person with dementia experiences is a result of the dementing process (Jones 2000). People with dementia are usually elderly and are likely to suffer from other acute and chronic illnesses which can increase confusion. Furthermore, the treatment given for such illnesses can, in itself, be a source of increased confusion in the elderly. Some commonly used drugs are known to be implicated in acute confusional states (delirium): benzodiazepines, tricyclic antidepressants, antiparkinsonian drugs, steroids and analgesics, among others.

Pharmacokinetic and pharmacodynamic factors will affect both efficacy and side-effect profiles of drugs. Pharmacokinetic changes with ageing include reduced hepatic and renal clearance, reduced hepatic metabolism, changes in absorption and reduction in plasma proteins; all these may have an effect on blood concentration of drugs. In addition, it is important to remember that elderly patients, particularly those with dementia, are far more likely to suffer concurrent illnesses which may influence plasma drug concentrations.

It is also very important to acknowledge that with normal ageing, and even more with dementia, there are neurochemical deficits (decreases in dopaminergic, noradrenergic, cholinergic and serotonergic neurones and/or neurotransmitters) that make older people with dementia far more likely to suffer adverse effects from a drug given the same blood concentration (Ballard *et al.* 2001). Therefore, the 'golden rule' of 'start low, go slow' regarding pharmacotherapy in elderly dementia patients is of particular relevance.

Polypharmacy (the use of multiple medication regimens) is common in old age, with four in five people over 75 taking at least one prescribed medicine, and 36 per cent taking four or more drugs (Department of Health 2001). The higher risk of concomitant diseases in older people increases the need for multiple medication regimens, increasing the risk of drug interactions and adverse drug reactions. Polypharmacy can also result in poor compliance, which can then add to the health problems already suffered. It is, therefore, of paramount importance to regularly review patients' medication in order to rationalize therapy and minimise polypharmacy.

Pharmacological treatments for behavioural and psychological symptoms in dementia (BPSD)

It is important to start this section by emphasizing the recommendations highlighted in the guidelines published by Scottish Intercollegiate Guidelines Network (SIGN) 1998 and currently under review, regarding interventions in the management of behavioural and psychological aspects of dementia: 'non-drug interventions should always be considered along with drug options before treatment is started'. Furthermore, we should ask ourselves whether the symptom is severe and persistent enough to need intervention. If it is, can an augmentation of the support package or environment, or a specific psychological intervention, resolve or substantially improve the situation? If this is applied with no desirable effect, does the symptom remain severe enough to merit a trial of pharmacotherapy?

In the context of rehabilitation, if drugs are used, the challenge will be to ameliorate the symptoms in order to maximize functioning without producing undesirable side effects that, on the other hand, can jeopardize our attempts to improve the quality of life of the person with dementia and their carers.

It is recognized that the majority of people with dementia will develop some degree of psychological and behavioural disturbances at some point during their illness. There have been several attempts to describe these signs and symptoms in a meaningful way. The Neuropsychiatric Inventory (NPI) (Cummings *et al.* 1994) is an increasingly popular instrument which uses the following headings in its 12 item (Nursing Home) version:

Psychological

- delusions
- hallucinations
- elation/euphoria
- depression/dysphoria
- anxiety
- disinhibition *

Behavioural

- agitation/aggression
- irritability/lability
- aberrant motor behaviour
- night-time behaviours **
- appetite/eating changes **
- apathy/indifference *

* items whose attribution to 'psychological' or 'behavioural' might be viewed as arbitrary.

** added for the nursing home version

The following are some pharmacological interventions used in treating some of the above symptoms.

Insomnia

Once again, before medication other approaches should be explored. So-called 'sleep hygiene' includes:

- having a regular bedtime routine
- using relaxation techniques (some suggest drops of lavender or camomile oil on the pillow)
- having a hot milky drink; avoiding tea, coffee and alcohol
- avoiding excessively warm or cold rooms
- taking moderate exercise and fresh air during the day.

But if insomnia persists and is distressing for both patient and carer, the use of short-term hypnotic treatment might be indicated. Examples of drugs commonly used include shorter acting benzodiazepines, such as lormetazepam or temazepam. Longer acting ones such as nitrazepam should generally not be used in older people because of the risk of accumulation and hangover effect. Non-benzodiazepine agents such as zopiclone, zolpidem or zaleplon may be tried. The hypnotic clomethiazole may be useful. It should be initiated cautiously since its half-life may be extended in older people (Bazire 2000) and toxicity may develop.

Anxiety and agitation

The SIGN guidelines (1998) advise that short courses of benzodiazepines may be needed. Shorter acting agents, such as lorazepam, are preferred, but smaller doses of intermediate-acting diazepam may be used with caution.

ANXIOLYTICS: NON-BENZODIAZEPINES

Some antidepressants can be effective in those suffering from anxiety and restlessness. The most useful agents are those with anxiolytic effects, such as SSRIs, or trazodone (Sultzer *et al.* 1997). There is evidence that buspirone may be a useful option for some individuals (Goa and Ward 1996).

Psychosis and aggression

The SIGN guidelines advise the use of antipsychotics only if there are serious symptoms, such as psychosis, or if there is a risk of serious emotional or physical danger. If psychosis is present (symptoms such as delusions and hallucinations), an antipsychotic (or neuroleptic) should be prescribed, as there is no other medication that is proven to be of benefit (Sultzer *et al.* 1997).

If antipsychotics are used in dementia the following guidelines should apply:

- 'Start low (sometimes extremely low), go slow.'
- Use short-term if possible and review regularly. Be aware of the potential effect on cognition (McShane *et al.* 1997).
- Avoid or use with extreme caution if dementia with Lewy bodies is suspected.
- Monitor for side effects, particularly akathisia, which is easily mistaken for increased agitation, leading to escalation of dose and development of a vicious circle.
- Avoid routine use of anticholinergic medication for neuroleptic side effects as these agents can also worsen cognitive function.

CONVENTIONAL ANTIPSYCHOTICS

The literature regarding conventional agents cites extrapyramidal side effects (EPSE) such as akathisia, parkinsonism, dystonia and tardive dyskinesia. Other potential side effects include: sedation, anticholinergic effects (constipation, blurred vision, confusion), postural hypotension, cardiac conduction defects and falls. A clinical issue that is of particular importance is dementia with co-occurring extrapyramidal disorders such as dementia with Lewy bodies, where occasional extraordinary sensitivity to conventional agents is seen. For all these reasons, atypical antipsychotics may have special utility in patients with dementia (Rosenquist, Tariot and Loy 2000).

ATYPICAL ANTIPSYCHOTICS

These agents may have possible advantages with regard to efficacy and toxicity compared to conventional antipsychotic drugs. None of these drugs is licensed for the treatment of BPSD but they are accepted by Old Age Psychiatrists in the UK as regular treatments and the Bolam principle would apply. Furthermore, some of these agents can be particularly useful in treating psychotic symptoms in conditions such as Parkinson's disease and, with extreme caution, in dementia with Lewy bodies because of the low incidence of EPSE.

Until very recently, risperidone has been widely used in BPSD as the bulk of the work in this field had been focused on this drug. It has been an attractive choice due to its tolerability and relatively low incidence of EPSE (mainly at doses below 1 mg daily). There is relatively little published evidence about the use of olanzapine in people with dementia but it has been widely used as well. However, on 9 March 2004 the Committee on Safety of Medicines (CSM) released expert advice recommending that both risperidone and olanzapine should not be used to treat behavioural symptoms in older people with dementia because of the increased risk of cardiovascular effects, in particular, stroke. The CSM took this decision after reviewing the available data from trials of these two drugs and considering other relevant evidence.

At the moment, the above CSM recommendation has not been extended to other atypical antipsychotics, such as quetiapine, amisulpiride and zotepine. There is no evidence to suggest that any of these drugs has clear advantages over any others although quetiapine seems to cause much less EPSE than other antipsychotics.

The pharmacological treatment of psychotic symptoms in people with dementia is proving very challenging. Very small doses of typical antipsychotics, while monitoring for side effects, might be needed. We might see use of other compounds such as cholinesterase inhibitors considered for the treatment of psychotic symptoms in dementia.

ANTICONVULSANTS AND MOOD STABILIZERS

There is some evidence on the use of these agents in patients with dementia, for behavioural disturbance throughout the range from agitation to aggression. Valproic acid (sodium valproate and, more commonly in the United States, valproate semisodium) and carbamazepine may be used alone or in combination with an antipsychotic drug. Lithium has not been proved to be very useful for agitation and may be difficult to use in older people with dementia, as adequate fluid intake is very important and regular blood monitoring is needed.

Depression

Depressive symptoms are very common in older people and the prevalence of depression in those with dementia is high. Depression can be a very disabling condition for both patient and carers. If identified and treated appropriately, depression can improve, leading to better functioning and, in turn, help the process of rehabilitation. Some of the symptoms to look out for include: low mood, apathy, tiredness, changes in sleep and appetite, loss of interest and restlessness.

Taking into account the few studies conducted in patients with dementia and depression, there is evidence that tricyclic antidepressants, SSRIs (Selective Sero-tonin Re-uptake Inhibitors) and moclobemide (a reversible inhibitor of monoamine oxidase type A) are all effective. However, SSRIs (particularly citalopram, fluoxetine and paroxetine) and moclobemide are much better toler-ated than tricyclics, which should be avoided in patients with already compromised cognitive function. After due consideration of concurrent physical illnesses, concomitant drug therapy and associated factors, antidepressants should be started at the lowest recommended dose for the elderly and titrated cautiously against both clinical response and side-effect profile. Porter and O'Brien (1998) suggest considering the following factors when selecting an antidepressant for an older person:

- history of response to a particular agent
- history of tolerance (or intolerance) to particular drugs
- type of depression (agitated/retarded)
- concomitant drug treatment and possible drug interactions
- compliance
- concurrent physical illness
- liability to particular side effects such as hypotension, cognitive impairment and sedation.

Specific drug treatments for dementia

In the context of rehabilitation of a person with dementia, a drug that can have a positive effect on memory deficits, behaviour and functioning is undoubtedly worth considering. If we bear in mind that dementia is a progressive illness with a gradual decline affecting memory, behaviour and activities of daily living, any pharmacological intervention that can at least delay this decline could be considered a success.

In the UK, there are four compounds licensed for the symptomatic treatment of Alzheimer's disease and I will discuss them in more detail in this section. It is important to emphasise that these drugs are not a cure but a treatment for the symptoms of Alzheimer's disease and that not everybody on these drugs will clearly benefit from them (around 50 to 60% will show some response). There are no other specific treatments licensed for other dementias, although the importance of managing vascular risk factors is more and more appreciated.

Acetylcholinesterase inhibitors (AChEis)

There are three preparations which are marketed for the symptomatic treatment of mild to moderate Alzheimer's disease: donepezil (Aricept®), rivastigmine (Exelon®) and galantamine (Reminyl®) (in the order they became available). Each drug is based on the cholinergic hypothesis of Alzheimer's disease which suggests that there is a deficit of choline acetyltransferase, the enzyme responsible for the synthesis of acetylcholine (a neurotransmitter implicated in cognitive processes), resulting in its reduced availability in the brain (Francis *et al.* 1999).

These compounds therefore increase cholinergic transmission between neurones by reducing the metabolism of acetylcholine, thereby increasing its availability. Each compound has a different chemical structure, relative reversibility and selectivity for cholinesterase; galantamine also enhances the action of acetylcholine on nicotinic receptors whereas rivastigmine also acts upon butylcholinesterase (an enzyme thought to be increased in Alzheimer's disease).

All three drugs have shown clear statistical and clinical advantage over placebo in terms of cognitive effects and behaviour (Wilkinson 2000) and also on activities of daily living. These changes, although somewhat modest, have been detected by both physicians and caregivers (Doody *et al.* 2001). A trial of three to six months is worth pursuing before deciding on the effectiveness of these drugs.

Although only licensed for mild to moderate Alzheimer's disease, there is increasing evidence that AChEis can be effective in the symptomatic treatment of other conditions such as dementia with Lewy bodies (Aarsland *et al.* 1999; McKeith *et al.* 2000). There have also been several studies suggesting that these drugs may be cost effective and can sometimes delay institutional care (Holmes *et al.* 1998; Small *et al.* 1998). After each of these drugs has shown clear benefits, some studies are now carrying out head to head comparisons between the different compounds.

Memantine

Memantine (Ebixa®) has recently been launched in the UK (October 2002) and it is the only drug licensed for the symptomatic treatment of moderate to severe Alzheimer's disease. Its mode of action is very different from that of AChE inhibitors, it modulates the glutamatergic neurotransmission system and is thought to act as a neuroprotector by preventing exposure of the brain cell to an excessive influx of calcium.

One study of patients with severe dementia has found that memantine leads to functional improvement and reduces care dependence (Winblad and Poritis 1999). Another study has shown reduced clinical deterioration in out-patients with moderate to severe Alzheimer's disease (Reisberg *et al.* 2003). A large randomized controlled trial looked into patients with mild to moderate vascular dementia and concluded that memantine improved cognition with no deterioration in global functioning and behaviour (Orgogozo *et al.* 2002). A recently published Cochrane Review (Areosa Sastre and Sherriff 2003) concluded that memantine was a safe drug and possibly useful in treating Alzheimer's, vascular and mixed dementia of all severities but that further studies were needed. As further comparative studies are carried out and if clinicians become able to treat their patients with memantine, clearer evidence of its benefits or otherwise will hopefully emerge.

Conclusions

Rehabilitation of a person with dementia, that is, maximizing potentials and minimizing disability, should start as soon as diagnosis is made. In this context, one of the main roles of the doctor as part of the multidisciplinary team is the rational use of medication. It is very important to acknowledge that older people, and especially those with dementia, are more susceptible to drug side-effects and drug interactions. We should, therefore, consider the following principles:

- 'start low, go slow'
- avoid polypharmacy when possible
- avoid medication that is likely to increase confusion
- use medication for BPSD only when necessary, when other approaches have failed.

Another duty of the doctor is to diagnose and treat any other physical or psychiatric disorder that the person with dementia might be suffering from.

The few specific symptomatic treatments for Alzheimer's disease that are available should be used. They are not a cure but in some people with dementia they can lead to an improvement in cognition, functioning and behaviour which, in turn, can facilitate rehabilitation, diminish carer distress and delay institutional care.

References

Aarsland, D., Bronnick, K. and Karlsen, K. (1999) 'Donepezil for dementia with Lewy bodies: A case study.' *International Journal of Geriatric Psychiatry 14*, 69–74.

Areosa Sastre, A. and Sherriff, F. (2003) 'Memantine for dementia (Cochrane Review).' *The Cochrane Library*, Issue 1, Oxford: Update Software.

Ballard, C.G., O'Brien, J., James, I. and Swann, A. (2001) *Dementia: Management of Behavioural and Psychological Symptoms*. Oxford: Oxford University Press.

Bazire, S. (2000) *Psychotropic Drug Directory, 2000*. Wiltshire: Mark Allen Publishing Ltd.

Cummings, J.L., Mega, M. Gray, K. Rosenberg-Thompson, D. and Gombien, T. (1994) 'The Neuropsychiatric Inventory: Comprehensive assessment of psychopathology in dementia.' *Neurology 44*, 2308–2314.

Department of Health (2001) *Implementing Medicines-related Aspects of the National Service Framework for Older People*. London: Department of Health.

Doody, R.S., Stevens, J.C., Beck, C., Dubinsky, R.M., Kaye, J.A., Gwyther, L., Mohs, R.C., Thal, L.J., Whitehouse, P.J., Dekosky, S.T. and Cummings, J.L. (2001) 'Practice parameter: Management of dementia (an evidence-based review). Report of the Quality Standards Committee of the American Academy of Neurology.' *Neurology 56*, 1154–1166.

Francis, P.T., Palmer, A.M., Snape, M. and Wilcok, G.K. (1999) 'The cholinergic hypothesis of Alzheimer's disease: A review of progress.' *Journal of Neurology, Neurosurgery and Psychiatry 66*, 137–147.

Goa, K. and Ward, A. (1996) 'Buspirone: A preliminary review of its pharmachological properties and therapeutic efficacy as an anxiolytic.' *Drugs 32*, 114–129.

Holmes, J., Pugner, K., Phillips, R. Dempsey, G. and Cayton, H. (1998) 'Managing Alzheimer's disease: The cost of care per patient.' *British Journal of Health Care Management 4*, 7, 332–337.

Jones, R. (2000) *Drug Treatment in Dementia* (1st edn). Oxford: Blackwell Science.

Jones, R. (2002) 'Rehabilitation.' In J.R.M. Copeland, M.T. Abou-Saleh and D.G. Blazer (eds) *Geriatric Psychiatry* (2nd edn). Chichester: John Wiley & Sons.

McKeith, I.G., Grace, J., Walker, Z., Byrne, E.J., Wilkinson, D., Stevens, T. and Perry, E.K. (2000) 'Rivastigmine in the treatment of dementia with Lewy bodies: Preliminary findings from an open trial.' *International Journal of Geriatric Psychiatry 15*, 387–392.

McShane, R., Keene, J., Gedling, K., Fairburn, C., Jacoby, R. and Hope, T. (1997) 'Do neuroleptic drugs hasten cognitive decline in dementia? Prospective study with necropsy follow up.' *British Medical Journal 314*, 266–270.

Orgogozo, J.M., Rigaud, A.S., Stoffer, A., Mobins, H.J. and Forette, F. (2002) 'Efficacy and safety of Memantine in patients with mild to moderate vascular dementia: A randomised, placebo-controlled trial (MMM300).' *Stroke 33*, 7, 1834–1839.

Porter, R.J. and O'Brien, J.T. (1998) 'SSRIs may well be best treatment for elderly depressed subjects.' *British Medical Journal 316*, 631.

Reisberg, B., Doody, R., Stoffler, A., Schmitt, F., Ferris, S. and Mobius, H.J. (2003) 'Memantine in moderate-to-severe Alzheimer's disease.' *The New England Journal of Medicine 348*, 1333–1341.

Rosenquist, K., Tariot, P. and Loy, R. (2000) 'Treatment for behavioural and psychological symptoms in Alzheimer's disease and other dementias.' In J. O'Brien, D. Ames and A. Burns (eds) *Dementia*. London: Arnold.

Scottish Intercollegiate Guidelines Network (1998) *Interventions in the Management of Behavioural and Psychological Aspects of Dementia: A National Clinical Guideline Recommended for Use in Scotland.* Edinburgh: SIGN 22.

Small, G.W., Donohue, J.A. and Brooks, R.L. (1998) 'An Economic Evaluation of Donepezil in the Treatment of Alzheimer's Disease.' *Clinical Therapeutics 20*, 4, 838–850.

Sultzer, D.L. *et al.* (1997) 'A double blind comparison of trazodone and haloperidol for treatment of agitation in patients with dementia.' *American Journal of Geriatric Psychiatry 5*, 1, 60–69.

Wilkinson, D. (2000) 'How effective are cholinergic therapies in improving cognition in Alzheimer's disease.' In J. O'Brien, D. Ames and A. Burns (eds) *Dementia*. London: Arnold.

Winblad, B. and Poritis, N. (1999) 'Memantine in severe dementia: Results of the 9M-BEST Study (benefit and efficacy in severely demented patients during treatment with memantine).' *International Journal of Geriatric Psychiatry 14*, 135–146.

CHAPTER 26

One Size Does Not Fit All: Person-centred Approaches to the Use of Assistive Technology

Stephen Wey

Introduction

Over the last five years I have been working as part of an intensive home treatment and rehab team for people with dementia. We work with people who would previously been likely to have been admitted to hospital for 'assessment' or who, having already been admitted, often for medical reasons such as falls or acute illness, find it hard to return to their own homes. Often there is a considerable degree of actual or perceived risk. In the course of these five years it has become apparent to me that not only has the pace of development of technological solutions such as assistive technologies increased rapidly, so too have their availability and the level of awareness of their potential benefits. There is still a long way to go, but I have no doubt that in the next few years occupational therapists will increasingly be finding themselves being asked 'Can you assess this person for a gas sensor?' in situations where previously they may have been asked 'Can you assess whether this person needs their gas cooker isolating?'. This has led me to ask some basic questions about why and when we would use such technology. I find myself asking not just where it would be useful and appropriate, but also where it would not be, or where it might in fact get in the way or cause more harm than good.

My starting point is that rather than mystifying the use of assistive technology by getting too hung up on its technical sophistication (and too often scaring ourselves off in the process), we need to get back to basics and understand it within the context of a process of rehabilitation. It seems to me that, whether we are assessing someone for and providing an 'easy-reach' or an 'intelligent' falls or gas detection system, the value system within which we operate and the underlying assessment and treatment process should be fundamentally the same. Our aim is to enable and empower that particular person and to help bring the world around them back within their grasp. We should not disable them by pushing the world further away or by making it harder for them to understand and control. We aim to improve their sense of agency and hope and their social confidence and self-esteem. We help them retain their personhood, their sense of who they are and of life having meaning, and of being valued persons in their own right.

As Mary Marshall has argued elsewhere, assistive technology '…is best seen as an extension of the aids and adaptations provision beyond static pieces of equipment' (1995). In the context of dementia rehab I would argue assistive technologies can potentially help:

- support and facilitate the person's memory, orientation and other cognitive abilities that are central to their everyday life
- enable the person to carry out tasks and activities that were becoming beyond, or in danger of becoming beyond, their reach
- facilitate meaningful occupation during the day, including leisure activities and maintenance of valued roles (such as participation in family life and social contact with friends)
- ensure the person's safety
- support and reassure carers.

However, like any form of aid or adaptation, the newer technologies are only tools employed for a specific purpose. A good analogy is the provision of specially adapted seating. Used appropriately such seating can and does facilitate people with postural impairment to achieve a higher quality of life. Used inappropriately, as we all know, such seating can serve as a form of restraint. Whether assistive technologies serve to enable or further disable the person depends therefore on the quality of the assessment process and particularly on how well the individual in question's own wishes and goals, their capabilities and their life history and social context are taken into account. These are things a person-centred approach to dementia rehab should base itself on; assessment for assistive technology cannot and should not be based primarily in a risk assessment, or even in an assessment of needs, but in a holistic assessment of the person's relationship with their social environment.

> Any failure to adequately consider the social context in which such technologies are placed might, therefore, result in the reinforcement of medical models of old age and service provision. (Fisk 2001)

One of the things I have tried to do recently is to reflect upon cases where the identified risks have been the same or similar but where the approach adopted has been different, in order to analyse the process of clinical reasoning behind each intervention. For example, many of the clients I work with have had problems with using cookers and continuing to cook for themselves. One major cause for concern is when people forget to turn the cooker off, leading to risk of fire or, if they have gas cookers, explosion. I have chosen three examples of people experiencing this problem and the identified intervention.

Mary

Mary was the first client with whom we tried using an assistive technology approach. She was a fiercely independent woman living alone. She had multi infarct dementia and, when referred to us, appeared to have recently undergone a 'stepwise' deterioration. She had been assessed by a community occupational therapist and was felt to be unsafe using her cooker and to need homecare to prepare meals for her. She had left the gas on several times, lit and unlit, and having her cooker disabled was being considered. One problem was that she was not willing to give up her cooking, which was an activity that was highly valued and an important aspect of her personhood. More practically she was not prepared to even let homecare in a lot of the time, let alone to do her cooking.

On further assessment it was noted that Mary was able to cook successfully 95 per cent of the time and was able to make quite complex dishes such as apple pies and meals involving several pans going at the same time. There were fluctuations in that level of competence, though, and it was during these periods that she was more at risk. Close observation of Mary carrying out activities like cooking and shopping showed that when functioning her best she was able to problem-solve well, carry out a number of aspects of the activity at once (multi-tasking), sequence the activity from beginning to end and maintain her attention on it even when doing other things like engaging in conversation. What was particularly noticeable was that procedural skills were very intact. She did well on a 'doing' level, even though her linguistic skills were highly impaired, leading to an impression that she was much more confused than her task performance indicated.

Mary seemed to have a few days every few weeks or so when her functioning would become compromised. Occasionally factors such as chest infections appeared to play a role in this, though not all the time. It was possible that she was also experiencing transient ischaemic attacks followed by increased confusion and then some recovery of function over subsequent days. (People like Mary are a good reason why intensive dementia rehabilitation is so essential, because if we can help facilitate that recovery and help them retain key skills and elements of their life roles and routines during these critical periods of remission we can help such individuals to continue to carry on their lives as they would wish to.) During these periods Mary would become highly distractible and have difficulty concentrating on what she was doing, she would be much more disoriented to time and place, her capacity to multi-task appeared to vanish, as did her problem-solving skills, which meant that she would be less able to recognize risk or know what to do in such situations. She was only able to sequence two to three stages of an activity at a time and would then lose the thread, and her speech would be more slurred and disjointed.

It seemed very unfair to be depriving Mary of such a valued activity and perhaps one that helped her recovery from periodic confusion by keeping her mind and body engaged in meaningful and validating occupation, for the sake of fluctuations in her confusion that only occurred 5 per cent of the time. It seemed better to enable her to continue to cook and, if anything, to help make the task more meaningful to her, while providing a relatively unobtrusive safety net in the form of a gas sensor that automatically shut off the gas if it reached a dangerous level. The fact that over the next few months this sensor went off less than a handful of times confirmed our initial assessment.

Clara

Clara was someone we helped return home from a medical ward. She had been admitted with a fractured neck of femur and had recovered well medically but was felt to be too confused and disoriented to go home. There were also concerns following a kitchen assessment on the ward about her safety preparing meals, as she had neglected to turn off the cooker and had difficulties sequencing what she was doing. The whole package of rehabilitation and the full role of assistive technology played in helping Clara to readjust to a return home is best discussed elsewhere, but the intervention used to enable her to continue to cook safely was relatively 'low tech' compared to Mary. When reassessed cooking in her own home, Clara proved to have pretty good problem-solving skills and was able to come up with creative solutions when presented with problems. She was aware of how to respond to risks appropriately and was provided with an alarm system. She was also able to sequence and to multi-task and once back at home was fully oriented to place (in contrast with the ward environment). She was able to concentrate and was largely non-distractible. She had some visual and auditory deficits that meant she had to put more into concentrating on the task in hand. At times this led to her not taking on board feedback from what she was doing; not noticing when something was not fully turned off, for example. This was not helped by the fact that the cooker was old and the markings on the dials were indistinct.

Once we had provided her with some stickers on the cooker clearly marking the on/off positions and provided her with a few clear written cues to ensure everything was off in strategic places she was able to cook light snacks (one pan dishes, toast, porridge) for herself safely. We also spent a couple of weeks working jointly with Clara in activities like cooking to help her build up her confidence and further assess her range of capabilities. Interventions and prompts were aimed at a level that gave her just enough support to carry out the activity without experiencing a sense of failure, but not so much that she felt we were taking over from her or invalidating her. At the end of this Clara decided that, while she wished to prepare her own snacks, she found more involved cooking a chore herself. So she was provided with homecare to do it. She was happy with that as she was also getting a lot out of having regular visitors. Since it was more important to Clara that she have time to herself to use as she chose than to be fully independent in everything this was a good balance for her. On the other hand, if homecare had been doing all meals for her she would have found this too intrusive. It would have taken away not so much a valued skill and role (as in Mary's case), more her freedom to live as she wanted and not be tied to other people's schedules. Maintaining some independence by cooking snacks was still important.

Norma

Norma was living alone in the community. She had been gradually deteriorating for a couple of years and this had largely gone on unnoticed so she had no support package. I was asked to assess urgently following a fire caused by Norma leaving a pan burning on the hob (luckily not a major one). I found Norma to be highly distractible and to have difficulty in particular concentrating on more than one thing at a time and tasks involving more than a couple of stages. She had some problem-solving skills: she was aware of how to respond to risks and turn off the cooker but only if there was nothing else distracting her. I noticed also that if she was presented with too much to do at once, too many challenges, she would just turn off and give up, even if it meant leaving a pan burning. Her belief in her abilities was low and the recent fire had made an impression on her sense of self efficacy too. Norma told me that she did not really like to cook that much and was not used to cooking full meals for herself, preferring to heat up soup and eat 'finger foods' that do not require preparation.

My view was that she needed to be helped to retain her sense of agency in performing tasks she could still manage as her self-esteem was becoming undermined by a constant sense of 'failure' in completing such tasks. It made sense to try and reduce the demands presented to her (Gitlin *et al.* 2001) when she attempted to make use of the cooker rather than just taking that away from her completely and getting homecare to do everything. Therefore the intervention for the cooker was to remove all but one of the knobs (leaving the most immediate to her) and arrange the surface of the cooker so she only had the one ring to focus attention on. She did not use the cooker that often (less than once a day) but a smoke alarm was provided as a further safety net.

Table 26.1 Summary of interventions for clients with problems using a cooker	
Identified risk – leaving cooker on and unattended	
Mary	Self isolating gas alarm
	Compensation for fluctuating risk while maintaining competencies and meaning of activity
Clara	Improve visual feedback and maintain competencies and confidence
Norma	Reduce demands of task
	Elimination of non essential distractions and streamlining of tasks
	Safety systems as backup

So if we start from the risk – the same risk in each case – we do not arrive at similar solutions (see Table 26.1). A detailed person-centred and occupational analysis focused assessment process shows that one size does not fit all. For each 'problem' there is a radically different solution or set of solutions depending on the individual, their social environment, their approach to activities and their life histories. For Mary a very new (at the time) piece of assistive technology was used to help her maintain her independence and personhood, whereas for Clara and Norma the interventions were more 'low tech' and in some respects more creative.

Conclusions

Like all social-technical change, the development of assistive technology brings both opportunities and threats. We need an approach that enables us to make the most of the opportunities it presents to form an important component of social support systems that help elderly people with dementia to live their lives the way they choose. This is what Fisk describes as 'Liberation technology' (Fisk 2001). The danger is that the agenda is allowed to be dominated by issues of risk and by achievements in the technical arena without fuller consideration of the human context. These are tools, no more, no less. It is the uses we choose to put them to that count. To sum up, in my view, provision of assistive technology needs to be seen within a rehabilitative and therapeutic context. It should:

- be based on an individual assessment of the person's capabilities, priorities and wishes – not just risk or need

- be based on an assessment of the way the person makes use of activity – that is the role such activities play in their lives, their meanings and routines

- aim to increase the fit between the person and environment (Rogers 1981), not decrease it (that is, it should bring the world more fully within the person's grasp, not make it more complicated or push it further away)

- enable the person to maintain a balance of occupations and social roles (such as leisure roles, carer roles)

- be meaningful to the individual; this means providing real choice, based on clear consent processes, sensitive to people's culture and life history.

In my view it is vitally important for practitioners to influence this developing agenda. We need to find ways to improve the dialogue and cross pollination between technologists, clinicians and service users to ensure that it develops in a direction that benefits the people who need it the most. Placing the assistive technology agenda within the context of a person-centred, social model of dementia rehabilitation is vital if we want to ensure that assistive technology is fitted to the individual, not the individual to the technology.

References

Fisk, M.J. (2001) 'The implications of smart home technologies.' In S.M. Peace and C. Holland *Inclusive Housing in an Ageing Society: Innovative Approaches.* Bristol: The Policy Press.

Gitlin, L.N., Corcoran, M., Winter, L., Boyce, A. and Hauck, W.W. (2001) 'A randomised controlled trial of a home environmental intervention: Effect on efficacy and upset in caregivers and on daily function of persons with dementia.' *The Gerontologist 41,* 1, 4–14.

Marshall, M. (1995) 'Technology is the shape of the future.' *Journal of Dementia Care 3,* 3, 12–14.

Rogers, J.C. (1981) 'The Issue is – gerontic occupational therapy.' *American Journal of Occupational Therapy 35,* 663–666.

PART SIX

Specific Difficulties

CHAPTER 27

Pain and Dementia

Jose Closs

Introduction

Older people make up a section of society whose pain has been largely ignored until recently. In general, pain management is poor among older people who do not have any cognitive impairment, and it may be far worse among those who have dementia or whose communication skills are otherwise compromised. However, with a little more knowledge and attention, unnecessary pain is something which can to a great extent be avoided.

Although painful conditions are not inevitable consequences of ageing, they certainly become more common as we get older. The prevalence of osteoarthritis, rheumatoid arthritis, back pain, cancer, pain with associated with stroke, vascular disease and peripheral neuropathies all increase with age. In parallel with this, the prevalence of dementia also becomes greater. As we get older therefore, there is an increasing chance of having both pain and dementia to varying extents.

It is clear that pain can reduce the quality of life, and that attention to the assessment of pain, its treatment, and evaluation of that treatment are crucial. Although all three of these stages of pain management are essential, it is the accurate assessment of pain which is key, since this is what drives successful treatment.

Pain reduces quality of life

If older people are allowed to endure pain unnecessarily, it can seriously reduce the quality of their lives. For example, it can have the following consequences:

1. It can make moving difficult. Those with arthritic joints, for example, become less mobile, and this can reduce their ability to look after themselves. It may be more difficult to get around and socialize, or

get to the bathroom unaided, or simply comb their own hair. Rehabilitation can be seriously hampered.

2.   It can cause or worsen depression and/or withdrawal. This is likely to reduce the motivation and ability to co-operate, again impeding rehabilitation. Their ability to maintain social integration may be reduced by negative moods.

3.   It can cause agitation. Those who cannot express their pain verbally may become frustrated at their inability to do so and become agitated as a result. For those with more severe dementia, it is possible that they may experience pain but are unable to recognize it as such, again producing agitated behaviour.

4.   It can interfere with sleep. Apart from the obvious problem of tiredness, the loss of sleep can increase fragmentation of usual patterns of rest and sleep, weakening overall circadian rhythmicity. This may then affect other aspects of behaviour which normally fit into a 24-hour cycle, causing or worsening temporal disorientation. Individually these negative effects of pain are undesirable, but together they may produce other problems. For example, if someone is tired, it hurts them to move and they are agitated, their risk of falling may be increased.

Issues to consider in the assessment of pain

There are three steps to consider in the management of pain: assessment, intervention and evaluation of the intervention. For those with dementia it is assessment which presents the greatest challenge. It is very difficult to work out how much pain is being experienced by someone who has profound dementia, although it is not usually problematic for those with mild to moderate cognitive impairment.

Methods of assessment

The assessment of pain can be undertaken very simply, and research has shown that those with mild to moderate dementia are usually able to give an accurate report of their own pain (Closs *et al.* 2004; Ferrell 1995; Parmelee, Smith and Katz 1993). It is mainly a matter of providing an opportunity for them to do so. This may begin with a general enquiry such as 'Have you got any pain or discomfort at all?' and if necessary, followed up with a simple intensity scale. The easiest scale to use and most successful for those with cognitive impairment is a simple verbal rating scale (Figure 27.1). This asks them to select which of the following words best describes their pain now: none, mild, moderate or severe. These words are best presented in large print (e.g. on a laminated A4 sheet) and read out at the same time, so the respondent can either give a verbal answer or point to the response they wish to give. Time and patience are needed, and the scale may need to be explained several times. However, there is a careful balance to be struck here – some may not be in enough pain to warrant completing the scale, and may resent too much persistence. Sensitivity and individualized knowledge of the person being assessed is needed.

Description of pain at this moment:

NONE

MILD

MODERATE

SEVERE

Figure 27.1 A simple verbal rating scale for pain assessment

Another simple scale is the numeric rating scale (Figure 27.2), which is a horizontal line with the numbers 0 to 10 spread equally across it from left to right, with 0 representing no pain and 10 representing the worst possible pain. Again, this should be explained patiently and presented visually in large print.

Description of pain at this moment:

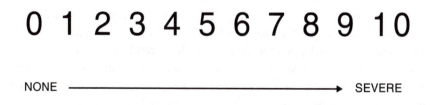

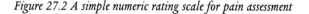

Figure 27.2 A simple numeric rating scale for pain assessment

Although those with dementia may have problems with their memory, they can usually give a reliable report of their pain at a given time. It is not a good idea to ask for retrospective pain reports, such as their worst pain over the previous 24 hours, since they may not remember. Ratings of pain given in response to assessments of current pain and the time at which these assessments were made should be recorded. It is important that assessments are then repeated, so that changes in pain level and the success of any pain control interventions can be identified.

Issues influencing pain assessment

There are many issues which may interfere with the straightforward assessment of pain (Table 27.1). Some are presented by the person in pain, some lie with friends and family, many are the responsibility of various health care professionals and some are the concern of all three groups (Cohen-Mansfield 2002; Furstenberg *et al.* 1998; Weiner and Rudy 2002). There is a wide range of factors that could interfere with the identification of pain and many of these are embedded in the knowledge and attitudes of formal and informal carers. They may not be aware of methods of assessing pain, they may not believe what they are told by the sufferer, they may assume no pain is present unless clear indications are volunteered by the sufferer and they may have exaggerated beliefs concerning the undesirable side-effects of analgesic drugs.

However, the greatest difficulties are with those who have severe cognitive impairment who may be unable to communicate their pain, verbally or otherwise. Although it is possible that their perceptions of pain are diminished due to the progressive deterioration of their brains, there is little evidence available to support this notion. Indeed, this is a dangerous assumption since there is no way of validating it convincingly and it may result in unnecessary suffering.

As has already been mentioned, self reports of pain intensity from those who have mild to moderate cognitive impairment have been shown to be as reliable as for those with no impairment, and should be believed. It has been suggested that the affective component of the pain experience (as opposed to its intensity alone) may be responsible for reduced reporting of pain in this group. There is, however, no clear support for this theory (e.g. Scherder and Bouma 1997). For this group it is important to rely on other evidence, such as the presence of an obviously painful condition (although back pain, headache, etc. will not be visible). Of vital importance is a knowledge of the history of the individual, and how they may have behaved when they were still able to express pain verbally. For example they may have indicated the presence of pain by rubbing the sore area, becoming silent and withdrawn, or becoming very noisy and agitated. Some preliminary work

Table 27.1: Issues to consider in the assessment of pain in older people with various levels of cognitive impairment

Person	Common issues
Older person	• from a generation which generally 'puts up with it' • often do not wish to complain and be seen as a nuisance • may not wish to acknowledge pain, since it may herald a serious disease and unpleasant treatment • may not wish to take any medications, because of fear of addiction, dependence or unpleasant side-effects • may not be able to use formal pain assessment instruments due to physical constraints (poor hearing or eyesight, motor impairments etc.) or mental constraints (depression and cognitive changes due to dementia) • may not use the actual word 'pain' when explaining how they feel, or be unable to express pain in words at all • may not be able to indicate pain non-verbally, by pointing, etc.
Formal carer (nurse, doctor, health care assistant, etc.)	• may believe that pain is a normal part of ageing • may not believe the person's report of pain • may not routinely assess pain in a structured way • may not know how to assess pain in people who have cognitive impairments • may not involve friends/family in assessing pain • may assume that little can be done to alleviate pain in older people • may be concerned about tolerance or addiction to analgesics • may confuse changes associated with ageing with painful conditions which may be reversed or treated • may not have enough staff/time to make this a priority • may be desensitized to the presence of pain • may not have access to relevant educational materials
Informal carer	• may not know about subtle manifestations of pain • may not have sufficient information about pain medications, their effects and side-effects • may be concerned about addiction to analgesics • may not wish to acknowledge pain since it may signify serious disease

has been done using facial expression (Hadjistavropoulos *et al.* 2002), but more work is needed to validate this and other behavioural approaches.

Pain control interventions

These are obviously crucial to successful pain relief, but for the most part may not need to be considered in relation to cognitive status, unless there is profound impairment. As for other groups, the provision of analgesic drugs is the main approach to pain control, with caution being exerted where there is genuine anxiety about the effects of drugs on cognitive functioning. It should also be remembered that there are changes in drug absorption, distribution, metabolism and excretion which occur as people age. Treatment may include opioid and non-opioid analgesic drugs or adjuvant analgesics, and these pharmacological approaches may be complemented by a range of non-pharmacological interventions. Pain specialists and multidisciplinary pain teams are increasing in number and have a significant role to play in identifying single or multiple interventions to suit individuals.

Pharmacological interventions

Analgesic drugs may be considered in three main categories. There are those which have a peripheral action, such as acetaminophen and non-steroidal anti-inflammatory drugs (NSAIDS); centrally acting opioid analgesics such as codeine and morphine; and adjuvant medications such as carbamazepine (primarily an anti-convulsant) and amitriptyline (primarily an anti-depressant). Adjuvants such as gabapentin are often helpful in the treatment of neuropathic pain. It is perhaps worth mentioning the relatively new class of NSAID here, namely coxibs, which have been found to be suitable for use with older people due to their superior safety in terms of gastro-intestinal and renal side-effects (see Lema 2003).

As a basic guide, the World Health Organization Analgesic ladder provides a validated instrument for providing pain relief for those with mild to severe pain. More general detail about analgesics for older people may be found in Abrahm (2000). A recent, simple scheme which 'incorporates the spirit of the WHO ladder' is the 'three-pot system' for acute and chronic pain relief (Bandolier 2003). This has been derived from the best available evidence and uses the least costly analgesic drugs. There are two different options, depending on whether or not the individual is able to take NSAIDs (Figure 27.3). This system maximizes the effectiveness of combinations of less potent analgesics, minimizing the number who may need to progress to stronger opioids such as morphine.

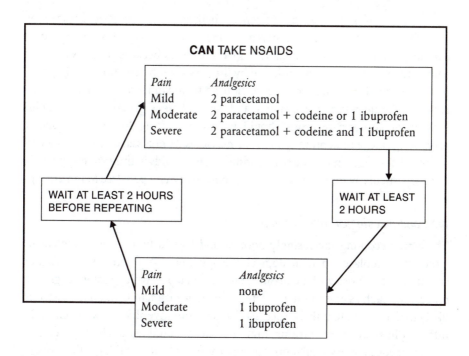

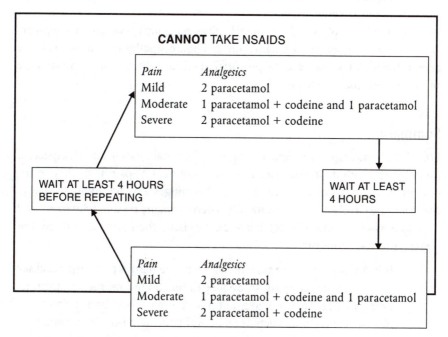

Figure 27.3 The three pot pain relief system (adapted from Bandolier 2003)

The presence of dementia may influence whether or not analgesic medications are either prescribed or administered. As mentioned earlier, those involved in pain management may be reluctant to give analgesics because they assume that pain is not present (not communicated by the person with dementia), or they may have concerns about respiratory depression, addiction or toxic side-effects. These concerns should not be exaggerated, and where there is genuine doubt, careful titration of appropriate drugs should be given, starting low and frequently reassessing and augmenting pain relief measures as necessary. It is difficult to obtain reliable figures, but the risk of addiction to opioids in this group appears to be tiny, particularly for those with chronic non-malignant pain (see Mann 2003).

Non-pharmacological interventions

These are becoming increasingly popular and should be used to complement rather than replace pharmacological therapy (see Allegrante 1996). Rather contentious for those with dementia would be therapies which require cognitive processing, such as education, relaxation, imagery, distraction and hypnosis. It is likely that these could only be successful where cognitive abilities were relatively intact. Physical interventions may be more suitable, such as exercise, transcutaneous nerve stimulation, the application of heat or cold, gentle massage and careful positioning.

It should be emphasized that the effectiveness of many complementary therapies, such as acupuncture, aromatherapy and homoeopathy, has not been clearly demonstrated, but some have the potential to create a distraction, and may have additional therapeutic effects.

Summary

Effective pain management then, is a big issue for rehabilitation and all aspects of care of those with dementia. The accurate assessment of pain is the key to the process of good pain management and this hinges on the ability either to communicate clearly or observe carefully. There are many reasons why pain is not accurately assessed, and although it is a complex issue, there are at least three clear messages to take from this.

1.   It is not acceptable to assume that someone has no pain, just because they don't (or can't) say so. Some painful conditions, such as arthritis or leg ulcer, may be obvious but others, such as low back pain or headache, may not. There is an ethical issue here since one cannot assume that someone has no pain just because they don't tell you about it. They may, of course, not have any pain, but it is quite likely

that they do. It would be safest to err on the side of caution and assume at least the prospect of pain, which might be confirmed by structured assessment, or perhaps the presence of pain associated behaviours.

2. Assess pain patiently and individually. Take a history of pain, its causes, related behaviours and previous successful approaches to controlling it. Involve family and friends if they feel able and willing to help. Understand that behaviours which are not obviously related to pain, such as agitation or withdrawal should be considered possible indicators and treated accordingly. Assess carefully and regularly. Re-assess once an intervention has had time to take effect. Consider additional approaches to analgesia if the first intervention is not effective.

3. Keep up to date with knowledge of methods of assessment and effective interventions. There are constant pharmacological developments, and those who prescribe for older people should keep abreast of these so that they may capitalize on analgesics such as coxibs. Similarly, evidence is regularly being produced concerning the effectiveness of complementary and other therapies, so that in future there may be scope for using more of these.

Conclusion

Quality of life may already be compromised in those who have dementia, and a little care and attention has the potential to produce considerable improvements in one key aspect of this, namely pain management. This can have a very positive impact on the lives of dementia sufferers, in terms of their mood, their ability to self-care and their ability to engage with others socially. It is up to us to do everything we can to minimize pain for those vulnerable people who suffer from dementia.

References

Abrahm, J.L. (2000) 'Advances in pain management for older adult patients.' *Clinics in Geriatric Medicine 16*, 2, 269–311.

Allegrante, J.P. (1996) 'The role of adjunctive therapy in the management of chronic nonmalignant pain.' *American Journal of Medicine 101*, (suppl 1A), 33S–39S.

Bandolier (2003) 'Easy targets aren't always the right ones.' www.jr2.ox.ac.uk/bandolier/painres/combos/comboed.html (accessed 30 June 2003). See also www.ebandolier.com

Closs, S.J., Barr, B., Briggs, M., Seers, K. and Cash, K. (2004) 'A comparison of five pain assessment scales for nursing home residents with varying degrees of cognitive impairment.' *Journal of Pain and Symptom Management 27*, 3, 196–205.

Cohen-Mansfield, J. (2002) 'Relatives' assessment of pain in cognitively impaired nursing home residents.' *Journal of Pain and Symptom Management 24*, 6, 562–571.

Ferrell, B.A. (1995) 'Pain evaluation and management in the nursing home.' *Annals of Internal Medicine 123*, 681.

Furstenberg, C.T., Ahles, T.A., Whedon, M.B., Pierce, K.L., Dolan, M., Roberts, L. and Silberfarb, P.M. (1998) 'Knowledge and attitudes of health-care providers toward cancer pain management: a comparison of physicians, nurses and pharmacists in the state of New Hampshire.' *Journal of Pain and Symptom Management 15*, 6, 335–349.

Hadjistavropoulos, T., LaChapelle, D.L., Hadjistavropoulos, H.D., Green, S. and Asmundsen, G.J. (2002) 'Using facial expressions to assess musculoskeletal pain in older persons.' *European Journal of Pain 6*, 3, 179–187.

Lema, M.J. (2003) 'Perspectives on pain management: The role of coxibs. Introduction: The role of coxibs in pain management.' *Journal of Pain and Symptom Management 25*, (2S), S3–S5.

Mann, E. (2003) 'Chronic pain and opioids: Dispelling myths and exploring the facts.' *Professional Nurse 18*, 7, 408–411.

Parmelee, P.A., Smith, B. and Katz, I.R. (1993) 'Pain complaints and cognitive status among elderly institution residents.' *Journal of the American Geriatrics Society 41*, 517–522.

Scherder, E.J.A. and Bouma, A. (1997) 'Is decreased use of analgesics in Alzheimer Disease due to a change in the affective component of pain?' *Alzheimer Disease and Associated Disorders 11*, 3, 171–174.

Weiner, D.K. and Rudy, T.E. (2002) 'Attitudinal barriers to effective treatment of persistent pain in nursing home residents.' *Journal of the American Geriatrics Society 50*, 2035–2040.

CHAPTER 28

Urinary Continence Rehabilitation in the Person with Dementia

Helen Leslie

There is a common belief among professional and lay people that incontinence is an inevitable part of ageing and that very little, if anything can be done (Wilson 2003). This view probably arises from the 'medicalisation of rehabilitation' (Oliver 1990). This 'medicalisation of rehabilitation' infers that the solution to all problems such as incontinence are to be found in medicine. However, the weakness of this view is that it ignores personal and social factors. An assumption is made that rehabilitation is about doing something to a person, for example prescribing medicines, and that when the medical intervention fails, nothing else can be done. Rehabilitation is much more about involving the person in exploring creative solutions to their problem. Rehabilitation has been defined as 'A process aiming to restore personal autonomy in those aspects of daily living considered most relevant by patients and service users, and their family carers' (Sinclair and Dickinson 1998).

For people with dementia the position is even more bleak, as it is often assumed that incontinence is the inevitable result of dementia, when in fact 'true loss-of-control incontinence of dementia should occur relatively late in the progress of the disorder' (Jacques and Jackson 2000). Incontinence in people with dementia before this late stage, then, should be investigated and treated and not assumed to be an inevitable part of dementia. Older people with dementia should experience equal access to investigation and treatment options as a person who is half their age.

Incontinence is estimated to affect between 43 and 62 per cent of residents in nursing homes (Conner and Lind 2001), which is a considerably higher rate than that of older people living in the community. Urinary incontinence is associated with skin problems, depression, social isolation and falls, and contributes to institutionalization in a number of older people. It has been suggested that the incidence of incontinence increases with the worsening of a person's mental state (Aggazzotti *et al.* 2000).

A continent person is able to recognize the need for the toilet, identify the correct place to meet this need and wait until it is socially convenient. An incontinent person may have a difficulty at any of these stages and rehabilitation must, as suggested by McGregor and Bell (1995), begin by a description of which part of the process is problematic. Causes of urinary incontinence may be urinary tract infection, constipation, stress incontinence, functional incontinence, bladder dysfunction, diuretic therapy and prostate enlargement. Functional incontinence results from cognitive or physical impairment, i.e. the person is unable to recognize the toilet, or unable to deal with clothing.

The first step in rehabilitation related to continence is that of assessment, in order to ascertain the cause of the incontinence and treat appropriately. The assessment process will include the completion of a fluid balance chart and a 'bladder' chart which will reveal patterns of incontinence. These charts should be maintained for seven days (Jones 1999).

It may be that a course of antibiotics or other medicine will rectify the situation. A change in diet may help. Urinary incontinence is often associated with constipation and therefore a diet high in fibre and with adequate fluids may rectify the problem. It would seem logical to reduce the amount of fluid a person takes if they are experiencing incontinence, but this in fact makes the problem worse. If fluid intake is decreased the urine becomes more concentrated, causes bladder irritation and therefore raises the likelihood of incontinence. However, altering the pattern of fluid intake may help with night time incontinence. If most of the fluid intake is before the evening meal, and the legs are raised in the latter part of the afternoon, which stimulates natural diuresis, less urine may be produced overnight (Conner and Lind 2001).

Stress incontinence may be helped by pelvic floor exercises. A person with dementia may need regular reminding about these, but commenced after an adequate assessment, the effect of these simple exercises can be dramatic.

> Mrs B had suffered from stress incontinence for about 20 years, which caused her to experience extreme social isolation. A nurse whom she had grown to trust persuaded her that the doctor might be able to offer help, and after a time she agreed. Her GP referred her for assessment, and from there she was referred to a physiotherapist specializing in continence issues. Within three months, as a result of perseverance with pelvic floor exercises, she was fully continent and began to participate in social activities.

Incontinence should always be investigated for physiological causes, and these physiological causes, if present, should be treated.

Routine

All of us have routines which help us to manage our lives, and a disturbance to these routines causes us stress. Compare the detail of your routine for the first hour of your day with the routine of a friend and imagine how you would feel if you were compelled to follow your friend's routine. Most of us have routines in relation to toileting, and to help a person remain continent for as long as possible, it is imperative that we find out as much detail as possible about their normal routine and then try to recreate that routine. This is not the same as having a two hourly toilet round – to be avoided at all costs – but assisting people to maintain continence in a person-centred way according to their own routine. Regular toileting can help 'reinstitute continence' (Jacques and Jackson 2000) by providing external cues to replace the lost internal cues.

The effect of the environment

One of the causes of people with dementia being admitted to long-term care is not true incontinence, though often described as such, but urinating in inappropriate places. This can be a source of much frustration for staff working in residential care, but some thought to a few design issues may resolve this situation. A major reason for this type of behaviour is that people with dementia are unable to recognize the whereabouts of the toilet, or even the toilet itself. In a communal living situation such as a care home, how do people recognize the toilet? Many signs on doors simply say the word toilet, which is not helpful if a person with dementia is no longer able to read or understand the meaning of words. There may be a picture of a man or a woman to denote male or female toilets, but often these symbols are not easy to recognize. Signage requires to be clear and easily understood. The word 'Toilet' and a clear picture of a toilet is probably the best combination (see Figure 28.1).

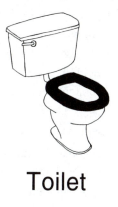

Toilet

Figure 28.1 Most easily understood toilet sign

However, understanding signs can be difficult for a person with dementia, and making the door itself easily recognizable is a good step. If all toilet doors in a building are the same distinctive colour, people with dementia will often come to recognize them whether signage is present or not. Painting the handrail the same distinctive colour helps people to find their way to a toilet door. Older people with dementia will not have accrued in their memory store a vision of a room with ivory tiles, and ivory toilet, an ivory toilet seat and beige flooring. They will have in their memory a white toilet with a black or dark brown seat. A toilet like this will not only be confirmed by their memory, but will also be visually clear.

> Mrs B entered Sunnyview, a specialized unit for people with dementia, where thought had been given to these issues. Toilet doors were rich burgundy colour, in marked contrast to other doors; they had clear signs and the toilets themselves were styled in a rather plain and old-fashioned way with black toilet seats. Mrs B had been living in a residential home and had moved to Sunnyview as a result of the difficulties caused by her using inappropriate places as a toilet, i.e. linen cupboards, blanket boxes etc.; her total refusal to sit on a toilet and her aggressive behaviour towards staff when they were required to intervene in her toileting. Doctors had been consulted and could offer no solution, staff at the residential home had tried to encourage her to wear pads which she refused. After two weeks at Sunnyview, with no particular intervention from staff, she was totally continent and using the toilet appropriately and independently. Staff could only conclude that this was a result of the toilets being designed to be recognizable to people with dementia.

There are other issues in relation to the environment that are likely to have an effect on continence.

- Rooms with ensuite toilets should be designed in such a way that the toilet can be seen from the bed if the door is open. If a person sees the toilet immediately on wakening it provides an extra cue, the person is not solely dependant on the sensation of a full bladder.

- Ensuite toilets should be lit with a low wattage light overnight. In the absence of ensuite toilets, corridors should be well lit.

- If at all possible toilets should be used in preference to commodes, particularly in shared accommodation. Screens may provide visual privacy, but do not provide privacy in relation to sound or smell.

- A means of calling for assistance should always be available.

- Handwashing after toileting may be encouraged if the hand basin is also styled in a more old-fashioned way, i.e. by the use of crosshead taps and a straightforward black plug on a chain.

As dementia advances, people can struggle to manage to remove clothing promptly enough to reach the toilet on time. One solution can be to suggest that easier to manage clothing is used, for example track suit trousers rather than tailored trousers. However, there is much more to clothing than body covering; the style of clothes that we wear communicates messages about ourselves and is closely linked to our sense of self, of who we are. As time passes and more of us have time for leisure, it may be that people will become equally comfortable in various clothing styles, but clothing style should remain firmly a matter of personal choice and should not be determined by issues like incontinence. In order that people can continue to wear their preferred style of clothing, adaptations can be made to make clothing easier and quicker to manage, for example, buttons and zips can be replaced by Velcro, stockings can be worn in preference to tights.

Continence rehabilitation for people with dementia requires a multi-faceted approach. Accurate and timeous assessment is the vital starting point. Physiological causes should be excluded, or treated if present. Consideration must be given to design issues. Clothing adaptations should be considered, if managing clothing is a problem. Routines need to be reviewed in a person-centred manner. Some or all of these interventions may help a person retain the dignity of remaining continent for a longer time.

References

Aggazzotti, G., Pesce, F., Grassi, D., Fantuzzi, G., Righi, E., De Vita, D., Santacroce, S. and Artibani, W. (2000) 'Prevalence of urinary incontinence among institutionalized patients: A cross-sectional epidemiologic study in a midsized city in northern Italy.' *Urology 56*, 245–249.

Conner, E.L. and Lind, L. (2001) 'Urinary incontinence in nursing homes: Epidemiology and Management Guidelines.' *Primary Care Update for Ob/Gyns 8*, 6, 248–252.

Jacques, A. and Jackson, G.A. (2000) *Understanding Dementia.* Edinburgh: Churchill Livingstone.

Jones, S. (1999) 'Promoting continence in older people.' *Elderly Care 11*, 8, 34–38.

McGregor, I. and Bell, J. (1995) 'A challenge to stage theories of dementia.' In T. Kitwood and S. Benson (eds) *The New Culture of Dementia Care.* London: Hawker Publications.

Oliver, M. (1990) *The Politics of Disablement.* London: Macmillan.

Sinclair, A. and Dickinson, E. (1998) *Effective Practice in Rehabilitation. The Evidence of Systematic Reviews.* London: Kings Fund.

Wilson, L. (2003) 'Continence and older people: The importance of functional assessment.' *Nursing Older People 15*, 4, 22–28.

CHAPTER 29

Dementia and Visual Impairment: Good Practice in Rehabilitation Work

Jim Crooks

Rehabilitation workers who are working with blind or partially sighted people in the community have a number of roles. They act as assessors, and are often required to assess within the framework of community care legislation. They provide training in daily living skills, Braille, typing and Moon, commonly referred to collectively as communication skills. Some workers will assess people for magnifiers to enhance the ability to read and write. Workers will also train people in independent mobility, which can range from a confidence building exercise and road safety work to a full course of training with a long cane. This can last for three months or longer and will involve ideally more than one session per week. Much of the work undertaken by the rehabilitation worker will be instructional and the underlying ethos of the profession is to maximize realistic independence for the client.

What will assist the worker to undertake these varied tasks effectively with a client with dementia? The question itself seems to present a contradiction in terms when the issue of rehabilitation is raised and the first thing that the worker may need to address may be his or her own attitude. According to Welsh and Blasch (1987)

> …whenever the mobility specialist does encounter a client whose visual loss is accompanied by other impairments, he (the specialist) might have a sense of hopelessness and futility. He may despair of being able to have an impact on the individual's ability to function more independently. This attitude, if it persists, can be the most serious impairment that the client has to overcome.

When dealing with dementia and visual impairment it is necessary for the worker to remember that it is the client who is the most important person in any relationship that needs to be formed. An intervention that can improve the quality of life as experienced by the client is a step forward, and small improvements can make a massive difference for certain individuals. Each individual is entitled to an assessment that takes into consideration his unique situation and is also entitled to an intervention that is tailored to his needs.

One of the most common tasks undertaken by a rehabilitation worker for the blind is to instruct a visually impaired client how to safely pour liquids. This enables people to prepare hot drinks for themselves. It is entirely possible that even although someone has memory problems they will be able to undertake a task like this for themselves. According to Rabinowitz (1986) 'cooking seems to be a skill that is retained in even moderately confused individuals'. The worker will need to make a judgement based on a sound assessment of the client's functional vision and level of consistent performance of the task. If clients can even pour for themselves it may allow a support worker to promote a level of activity that will afford some dignity and independence not previously available to the client. How much better might some people feel about their situation if they were able to make a simple meal for themselves or a sandwich and a cup of tea, if reminded where the necessary utensils were? It is essential for the rehabilitation worker to take a positive attitude to each individual and to the potential importance of the tasks they might undertake when a diagnosis of dementia is present. According to Welsh and Blasch 'the specialist must discipline himself to focus on abilities and potential as a necessary step toward helping the client reach that potential' (1987).

Joint working with other professionals and family members is an essential component of good practice, along with a positive attitude. This is nowhere more critical than in the assessment process itself. Although the main focus of rehabilitation worker training is on instruction, workers can be required to assess in the context of community care and in some cases to act as care managers. It may be that they are the first point of contact for a client and their carers with their local agency. In this case the issue of client risk is a significant one. While workers are trained to make judgements about risk relating to functional vision they are not qualified to make judgements about dementia and in this area it is important that they take advice from other professionals before making any decisions that may affect the client.

Rehabilitation workers are less frequently presented with crisis situations than social workers who are called upon to deal with these on a regular basis, yet when dealing with a client with dementia as a first point of contact a worker may be faced with a high risk situation and experience a level of stress and uncertainty.

Moore (1996) asserts that

...one of the most common weaknesses identified in risk assessment is the tendency for it to be carried out by a single discipline, or indeed individual. Accuracy is likely to be compromised as a result. In such cases it is the front line practitioners who are likely to be held responsible when predictions about risk fall short. They therefore have the most to gain by maintaining the pressure to improve inter agency cooperation. In each assessment where the need for outside/specialist input is identified, the assessor should declare this clearly and state how their own predictions have been compromised by this lack of input.

As the caring professions are moving towards what is described as 'joint working' and the process of 'single shared assessment' it is important for rehabilitation workers to realize that they are not alone when it comes to accountability and there may be a need for them to refer on to a psycho geriatrician, a social worker, or a GP for a further assessment when issues relating to risk are unclear.

According to Jacques and Jackson (2000) assessment should be 'assessment for a purpose' and 'we should always question the time and energy that is spent on assessment rather than on doing things with the patient'. It is the role of the rehabilitation worker to assess functional vision and to differentiate between problems arising from vision and problems arising from other areas or disabilities, and to work with problems related to loss of vision. Workers would wish to undertake training with the client in order to maximize realistic independence as a result of assessment.

Joint working with carers and other professionals is essential when the assessment results in training. Training can include help with orientation and mobility, daily living skills and communication. It will involve working with the client to improve skills in these areas. In addition to taking into account the element of risk, the assessment process is for the purpose of indicating what training should take place, how appropriate the training is and how it can be taken forward. In this case it is desirable for the worker to establish both what the client could achieve prior to losing their sight and what they would like to achieve at the time of assessment. In the case of dementia 'Background information gives the essential baseline in assessing what support the patient can expect from family and friends, what interests and activities she might continue to engage in and what her living conditions are' (Jacques and Jackson 2000).

When working with people who have additional disabilities and especially communication deficits it is essential to consult with those people who have a knowledge of the client's history so that a realistic plan can be made, implemented and supported. It is necessary when working in the community to establish links with the family and other carers in order to support training programmes for people who cannot learn quickly. This is because the pressure of waiting lists and the need to ensure that there is a throughput of clients does not allow workers the luxury of spending as much time as it might take to personally instruct a client, where progress can only be made through a considerable amount of repetition. Workers do not have unlimited time available for training when a positive outcome is dependent on many months or years of input. This does not mean that instruction cannot take place if there is a family member or a care worker who can reinforce learning. The worker can initiate training with the client and then hand the re-inforcement of learning over to someone else when repetition is necessary to fully integrate the skills being taught. This means working closely both with the client and the carer so that both have a clear understanding of the specific aims of training and how these are to be achieved in a practical sense.

Precision is necessary in this area so that there can be no confusion between the trainer and the support worker. If, for example, the client is learning the route from the living room chair to the toilet, both the client and the support person will need to know the exact sequence of landmarks that the client will have to locate to aid navigation, and if there are difficulties, the manner in which they can be located in space. In the case of difficulties experienced by the client the support person can communicate them to the rehabilitation worker, who may be able to suggest solutions. In an ideal world the rehabilitation worker would be able to establish a relationship with the client, which could in itself assist in providing motivation, and deliver the training themselves. Staffing and resources are not normally available to allow this in every case and managers are continually faced with the problem of allocating workers' time appropriately. There can be, however, positive advantages for someone with dementia in being supported by someone that they already know and recognize.

What instructional techniques are available to workers who are dealing with clients with dementia? When working with blind or partially sighted people it is important to maintain a consistent environment so that things are *always* kept in the same place. This means that they do not trip over unexpected obstacles or eat tins of dog food instead of beans. Maintaining a level of consistency in both the environment and the instruction will assist in establishing a positive outcome in terms of daily living skills and mobility. This will be doubly important for someone who is confused as well as blind or partially sighted.

Another feature of working with blind people is the breaking down of tasks of daily living into small units in order to deliver instruction, or making a 'task analysis' of such activities. This means that instructions are more manageable for the recipient. Clearly, for example, when spreading butter on bread a sighted person will not need to locate the knife and the bread, because doing that visually is taken for granted. When teaching a blind person each of those actions will be the subject of separate and clear instructions.

According to Davis, writing about people with dementia, 'the keys to teaching them include the use of one stage requests, followed by appropriate pauses to let the request register' (1986) and it can be seen that there is a parallel between this type of instruction and the work undertaken by a rehabilitation worker in preparing a task analysis and using that for instruction. In working with people with dementia workers need to be aware of the importance of this type of instructional technique.

Another important factor in delivering instruction is preparing a suitable environment. It is important that distractions are kept to a minimum and that noise is not allowed to interfere with the learning process. It would seem obvious that this could be beneficial in most learning situations, but it is doubly important in dealing with people who are confused. Davis points out 'that sensory overload or an increase in the number or complexity of demands on Alzheimer's victims will frustrate them' (1986). This 'sensory overload' is increased if there is noise or multiple conversations occurring.

The majority of people registered as blind or partially sighted have some useful vision and for them some form of labelling (Davis 1986) or colour coding is useful as a prompt or a reminder for people with dementia. Rehabilitation workers are used to the idea of colour contrast as a way of picking out detail in the environment and this can be combined with a system that prompts memory. Labels can be colour coded also. In addition to the uses of colour for contrast rehabilitation workers need to be aware of the use of colour as an aid to memory.

It is also important to avoid negative reinforcers in training someone with dementia because this can be misinterpreted by someone with deficits in understanding. According to Pryor 'every instance of their use contains a punisher' (1985) and the severity of the punisher is open to interpretation. This can result in 'all the unpredictable fallout of punishment: avoidance, secrecy, fear, confusion, passivity, and reduced initiative, as well as spill over associations, in which everything that happens to be around, including the trainer and the training environment becomes distasteful or disliked, something to be avoided or even fled from' (Pryor 1985).

Good practice then, for the rehabilitation worker is dependent on a positive attitude to the likelihood of achieving a good result with the client; joint working with the client, the carers and other professionals throughout the process of assessment and provision; and the application of appropriately selected instructional techniques, some of which are familiar to rehabilitation workers already.

References

Davis, C.M. (1986) 'The role of the physical and occupational therapist in caring for the victim of Alzheimer's Disease.' In E.D. Taira (ed) *Therapeutic Interventions for the Person with Dementia*. London: Haworth Press.

Jacques, A. and Jackson, G.A. (2000) *Understanding Dementia* (3rd edn). London: Harcourt.

Moore, B. (1996) *Risk Assessment: A Practitioner's Guide to Predicting Harmful Behaviour*. London: Whiting and Birch.

Pryor, K. (1985) *Don't Shoot the Dog*. London: Bantam Books.

Rabinowitz, E. (1986) 'Daycare and Alzheimer's Disease: A weekend programme in New York City.' In E.D. Taira (ed) *Therapeutic Interventions for the Person with Dementia*. London: Haworth Press.

Welsh, R.L. and Blasch, B.B. (1987) *Foundations of Orientation and Mobility*. New York: American Foundation for the Blind.

PART SEVEN

Conclusion

CHAPTER 30

Learning about Rehabilitation and Dementia from Many Perspectives

Mary Marshall

The journey through this book has not been a linear one, indeed the term 'radiant' used by the mind mappers (Buzan and Buzan 2000) would be appropriate in that the authors have woven a rich, complex, multi-layered web of this concept. Starting from rehabilitation, they have branched out in many different but overlapping directions. The contributions from people with dementia and their families (Susan Fleming, Morris Friedell, Tom and Sheila Davis and members of the PROP group) provide the central core of this web and anchor it firmly in reality. Almost all the authors point out that the use of the term 'rehabilitation' alongside 'dementia' is an unusual one, to be welcomed.

Take the *focus* of rehabilitation as one dimension in this web. For people with dementia it is on the dementia itself, for Peter Murdoch it is on the impaired functioning resulting from an injury or episode of illness, for Barry Wiggins and Jenny Fahy it is food, drugs and social support, for Joy Harris it is communication and language. Helen Leslie was specifically asked to write about incontinence since I surmised, rightly, that it would not be mentioned unless I organized some input. This is surprising given the extent to which it affects people's self-image and confidence. I also asked Cesar Rodriguez to address medication issues in order to ensure these are well covered. David Jolley, like many others, emphasizes the importance of a focus on relatives and carers. Many of the authors focus on self-esteem and confidence. This can be eroded when you get dementia and this erosion can be exacerbated by care settings. Susan Nixon describes how a Norwegian home gave every resident a role in order to counter this. Faith Gibson suggests that life story work is another approach to address these losses.

This book is probably unique in collecting so many different professional and personal perspectives. Sarah Rhynas is the most explicit about her profession of nursing conceptualizing the term rehabilitation in both functional and social terms, yet the different ways it is conceptualized is implicit in all the papers. The same is true of dementia. David Jolley's chapter shows the way dementia is conceptualized by a psychiatrist. This self-awareness is important since one of the problems is that many people do not know what they do not know, and they need to be given the necessary knowledge and skills. The short papers in this book should lead readers to the references and to more extensive reading. It is not, and was not intended to be, a manual about practice.

Most authors mention the need for *teamwork*. Carolyn Marshall's chapter is specifically about a team in which roles overlap without anguish about who does what. Ken Barlow is concerned that professionals such as occupational therapists, CPNs and social workers who struggle to describe what they do, will have their unique identity blurred by being 'reduced to a generic, nondescript dementia care worker'. Larissa Kempenhaar, Sarah Rhynas and Jim Crookes point out that it is the people who spend most time with the person, nurses and relatives, who have to implement and maintain the guidance of the professional teams. Peter Murdoch includes the family in his consideration of teamwork. Jim Crookes writes from the perspective of a rehabilitation team for visually impaired people, some of whom have dementia. He is insistent that this is only possible if workers are clear that they are not alone; there is a host of other professionals to assist.

One of the differences between authors is *where* the rehabilitation takes place. Both Barry Wiggins and Carolyn Marshall work in the community. Peter Murdoch suggests that there must be interventions in the community, which prevent hospital admissions. There are different perspectives on specialist services. Susan Nixon describes what can be offered in a specialist care home. Kate Read and Sarah Rhynas both acknowledge the value of specialist units but feel that this care needs to be rolled out into non-specialist settings. Kate Read also pleads for more effort to involve primary care. Ian Greaves is the only author, perhaps understandably, who mentions primary care as a setting for a range of sorts of help including consultations with consultant psycho-geriatricians and special workers (who have to be bribed with coffee!).

In the first chapter I reflected on the fact that *time* was probably a critical issue and this is borne out by many contributions. Peter Murdoch points to the evidence that people with dementia do appear to benefit from rehabilitation after acute illness, although it may take longer. Barry Wiggins and Jenny Fahy report their staff can spend weeks gaining the trust of people with dementia living at home. They provide case studies to reinforce this point, as do Carolyn Marshall and Allison Black. Susan Nixon suggests that time, or lack of it, may be the reason why people with dementia fail to receive rehabilitation in acute hospital wards. Like many authors, she also draws attention to Nolan's (2001) two models of rehabilitation, one highly specific and time-limited and one comprehensive and long term. This is probably the same differentiation as that between rehabilitation as an intervention and rehabilitation as an approach, which underlines a lot of the contributions. Many of the contributors are describing an approach with a strong value base, emphasizing the importance of seeing the whole person with a history, in a context, and for whom there is always something that can be done. Christine Davidson and Claire Black recognize that what can be achieved may be only a period of fun and enjoyment.

Many contributors have resisted the potentially mechanistic temptation to talk about the *stages* of dementia and what can be expected at each stage. They have instead opted for a highly individualized approach avoiding any preconceptions resulting from knowledge of the stage of dementia alone. Stephen Wey's contribution typifies this approach in its attention to competence and individual preferences rather than the stage of dementia. This is probably because they are all experts with a lot of experience, who know the clinical aspects sufficiently well that they feel their priority must be a focus on the many other factors which affect the experience of dementia. This may be less helpful for someone new to dementia care. David Jolley's paper is especially useful for these readers. He is not alone in mentioning the different approaches at different stages. Linda Claire is clear that cognitive rehabilitation is more effective in the earlier stages. Jose Closs too refers to different stages of dementia when he is talking about pain. He suggests that people in the mild to moderate stages can give an account of pain but, later on, it may depend on staff and relatives having a knowledge of the individual and how they expressed pain in the past. Ian Greaves' view on stages is the failure of many GPs to diagnose and offer help early enough.

Learning and motivation are, as I said in the introduction, usually assumed to be required for rehabilitation, yet these are problematic for people with dementia. Larissa Kempenhaar specifically addresses this issue 'where in mainstream physiotherapy patients are expected to remember exercises, advice and previous treatments, this may not be possible in dementia rehabilitation'. She goes on to make several suggestions of ways to get round this problem. Morris Friedell tells us just how problematic these skills are and offers us six steps he has developed for people with dementia to work on their own rehabilitation. Adjusting to changes in ability is usually seen as part of the rehabilitation process and the PROP group participants show how much a group can help with this. The two speech therapists also work with groups and show how useful this kind of intervention can be. Most other contributors describe interventions with individuals and with families.

Cognitive rehabilitation specifically addresses the issue of *learning* when you have dementia. Linda Claire is clear that despite difficulties with memory and other functions, 'people with dementia still have the ability to learn new associations and information to adjust their behaviour and responses'. She emphasizes the aim of strengthening the sense of self and identity and enhancing feelings of being in control. Although the authors may not describe their work as cognitive rehabilitation, much of the work described in the chapters has the same aim. Being in control impacts fundamentally on motivation. Stephen Wey, for example, talks about using technology 'to enable and empower…to bring the world around them back within their grasp'; in my chapter about the environment I suggest that 'stress is reduced if people feel, in some way, in control of their environment'. Maria Parsons claims that the contribution of social work is to enable the person with dementia to achieve maximum control and choice.

Gail Mountain's literature review demonstrates how many aspects there are to rehabilitation and dementia. She shows how little research evidence there is for most *interventions* and how much work remains to be done. However, she also identifies areas where an evidence base is beginning to exist. We should not be surprised that there is such patchy evidence given the challenge of mapping the field: until it is described and defined it is not easy to do the necessary research.

The rich, complex and multi-layered web this book has woven reflects the current reality of dementia care. I began this book with a description of four approaches to our understanding of dementia. This book reflects these four approaches, especially the need to have the person with dementia recognized as a unique individual. People with dementia have also made their own contributions in this book to our understanding of dementia and of rehabilitation. Suzanne Cahill and Avril Dooley's brief account of the history of the concept of rehabilitation shows how it is not a static concept: it too has widened and deepened.

Rehabilitation and dementia are both developing worlds and it should not surprise us that it is difficult to come up with clear definitions and clear practice guidance. This book will undoubtedly sensitize professionals, planners, managers and commissioners to the potential of rehabilitation with people with dementia. It will also alert them to the need for lateral thinking and creative approaches. The book has provided a lot of examples as well as further reading. It must, however, be seen as 'work in progress' rather than any sort of final document on the subject.

References

Buzan, T. and Buzan, B. (2000) *The Mind Map Book*. London: BBC Worldwide Ltd.

Nolan, M. (2001) 'Acute and rehabilitative care for older people.' In M. Nolan, S. Davies and G. Grant (eds) *Working with Older People and their Families. Key Issues in Policy and Practice*. Buckingham: Open University Press.

Contributors

Ken Barlow trained in Newcastle-upon-Tyne in the early 1970s followed by various posts in hospital and community settings in north-east and north-west England. He was Nurse Tutor to the CPN Cert course and then P2000 in Newcastle-upon-Tyne before returning to clinical practice in Scotland in 1996.

He is currently working as CPN in a multi-disciplinary community mental health team for elderly people in Dumfries and Galloway whilst concurrently studying for a Post-graduate Dip/MSc in Dementia Studies at the University of Stirling, Scotland.

Rona Bissell works for a Community Mental Health Team for Older People in Dundee. She graduated from the Glasgow School of Occupational Therapy in 1991, and has worked in the psychiatry of old age since graduating in organic and functional illness. She has worked in admission wards, rehab, long stay and day hospital, with a particular interest in organic illness and functional assessment.

Allison Black is a registered mental nurse and worked with the Central Aberdeenshire Community Dementia Team from 1992 to 2003. She was employed by Grampian Primary Health Care as a nursing nightsettler until 2000 and as support worker supervisor and acting care manager from 2000 to 2003.

Claire Black is a speech and language therapist in dementia care working with an in-patient caseload. She has been in her present post for five years.

Suzanne Cahill is the Director of Dementia Services Information and Development Centre Dublin based at St James Hospital and a Lecturer in Gerontology in Trinity College Dublin. She comes with a background in social work practice, teaching and research. She wrote her PhD on the topic of aged care policy, dementia and family caregiving and has published widely in this area. Her current research interests include, dementia and quality standards, women and social policy, family caregiving, assistive technologies and dementia and elder abuse.

Linda Clare is Lecturer in Psychology, University College, London, and Consultant Clinical Psychologist, Camden and Islington Mental Health and Social Care NHS Trust. She is a clinical psychologist and neuropsychologist specializing in dementia research and rehabilitative work with people who have cognitive impairments arising from dementia and other age-related conditions. Recent research has included the development of cognitive rehabilitation interventions for people with early-stage dementia. As well as publishing numerous journal articles, she has co-authored a book on coping with memory problems and co-edited a volume on cognitive rehabilitation in dementia, and is on the editorial board of the journal *Neuropsychological Rehabilitation*.

Jose Closs is Professor of Nursing Research in the School of Healthcare Studies, University of Leeds. She has been involved in clinical nursing research for two decades, and has become increasingly interested in pain management in recent years. Of particular interest are gaps in care provision, in particular for groups who do not have a 'voice', such as older people and in particular those who have difficulty in communicating their pain.

Jim Crooks has been working with visually impaired people for 12 years. He works for a national charity in Edinburgh managing a team of rehabilitation workers. He is qualified in rehabilitation and social work, and is a graduate of both Aberdeen and the Robert Gordon University.

Christine Davidson is a senior occupational therapist working for Tayside Primary Care NHS Trust. Christine graduated from the University of Northumbria in 1995 and has worked in a variety of community and hospital settings with older people who have mental health problems since then. Special interests include occupational science and the use of activity in promoting communication, personhood and, of course, independence.

Sheila Davis is 81 years old. She spent seven years in the Wrens during World War Two honing the culinary skills that later in life were to 'delight' her five children. Sheila was also a foster mother to countless other babies in the Manchester/Salford area during the 1950s and 1960s. She was diagnosed with dementia in 2003. Sheila uses her indefatigable sense of humour and the support of Tom to continue to enjoy life.

Tom Davis is 79 years young. Tom served in the Pacific in the RAF during World War Two. He returned to his native Bolton where he worked his way up from plumber's apprentice to running his own businesses on Tyneside. Now retired, Tom enjoys bowling and playing bridge. He is a very committed carer and husband. Tom means to honour his wedding vows of 'for better for worse, in sickness and in health' for as long as he is able.

Avril Dooley holds a Masters degree from Trinity College Dublin in Applied Social Research. She was employed as a Research Assistant at the Dementia Services Information and Development Centre, Dublin in 2003 when she wrote her Masters thesis on the topic of the role and benefits of meaningful activities for people with dementia resident in nursing homes.

Susan Fleming works as a project worker with the Joint Dementia Initiative in Falkirk.

Morris Friedell was a Professor of Sociology at the University of California, Santa Barbara. He taught a course on human dignity in which the human potential for heroism in adversity was explored, never dreaming that this background would one day help him face the challenge of Alzheimer's.

Faith Gibson is a graduate of the Universities of Sydney, Queensland and Chicago in social work and education. She is an Emeritus Professor of Social Work, University of Ulster. Her interests include various aspects of dementia care and service provision, and using people's past to sustain relationships and enhance communication in the present.

Ian Greaves is a general practitioner in a rural, teaching, first wave PMS plus practice at Gnosall, Stafford in the West Midlands of England. He has a list size of 7200 patients. He is honorary Senior Lecturer at Wolverhampton University and has a special interest in care of the elderly and managing dementia in the community. The practice is renowned for innovation and has won many national and international awards, culminating in being a finalist in the Department of Health 'Outstanding Achievers' awards 2003 for their contribution to innovation in service delivery over the past 20 years.

Joy Harris is the Mental Health Team Lead Speech and Language Therapist in East and Midlothian. She has worked in the field of mental health since 1995 and part of her remit is with the Dementia Team. She is also currently doing a post graduate diploma in counselling.

David Jolley is Director of Dementia Plus, Consultant Old Age Psychiatrist, Wolverhampton City PCT, and Professor of Old Age Psychiatry, University of Wolverhampton. A pioneer 'psychogeriatrician' in the north-west of England, establishing the first service in South Manchester 1975, Professor Jolley is active in service development, teaching, training and research. He was Chairman of the RCPsych. Section (now Faculty) of Old Age 1990–1994. He relocated to the West Midlands in 1995, developing community and mental health services in Wolverhampton, links to Wolverhampton University and the establishment of Dementia Plus.

His recent initiatives include the fight against 'post-code' prescribing; multi-disciplinary training; links with primary care; issues in residential care; stress in the work force; potential of physician assistants for the NHS and services for 'graduates'.

Larissa Kempenaar works as a Lecturer in Physiotherapy in the School of Health and Social Care at Glasgow Caledonian University. She developed an interest in dementia care while working in elderly mental health in Ailsa Hospital. There she was involved in several research projects investigating the effects of sensory stimulation on people with dementia and the effects of carer education on carers' levels of stress and depression. She is currently undertaking a PhD investigating carers' levels of stress and how these are influenced by the carers' control beliefs.

Helen Leslie is Education Manager for Carrick Care Homes and has just completed the MSc in Dementia Studies at the DSDC at Stirling University. Particular areas of interest in relation to dementia are autonomy, quality of life and relationships.

Carolyn Marshall is a senior social worker and Mental Health Officer for Aberdeenshire Council social work service. She has worked with Central Aberdeenshire Community Dementia Team for eight years as a social worker/care manager and since 2000 as Team Co-ordinator.

Mary Marshall has worked with older people as a social worker, researcher and teacher since 1974. She was the Director of Age Concern Scotland between 1983 and 1989 when she took the post of Director of the Dementia Services Development Centre at the University of Stirling. She is the author of numerous books, chapters and articles about work with older people and people with dementia. In 1998 she was awarded the OBE, and she was a member of the Royal Commission on Long Term Care of the Elderly. The Dementia Services Development Centre exists to extend and improve services for people with dementia and their carers.

Gail Mountain is an occupational therapist with experience spanning practice, management and research. Gail's research interests are concerned with research into rehabilitation services and interventions with older people. She is currently working as Head of Research in the School of Health and Social Care, Sheffield Hallam University, where she is responsible for fostering research across nursing, allied health and social work. Prior to this, Gail worked as research and development officer for the College of Occupational Therapists. She has also held research posts at the Universities of Leeds and York.

Peter Murdoch has been a consultant physician in geriatric medicine at Falkirk Royal Infirmary since 1983. He has a longstanding interest in dementia, helping to establish the Dementia Services Development Trust and DSDC in 1988, and has been a trustee since then, chairing the British Geriatrics Society / Royal College of Psychiatrists Joint Liaison Committee 1989–91, and has recently developed dementia care pathways for acute patients in his local district general hospital.

Susan Nixon is trained in social work and since qualifying her work has been almost exclusively with older people in residential care, including the management of a specialist care home for older people with dementia. She has recently completed the Post Qualifying Diploma in Dementia Studies at Stirling University, and is currently on a secondment that involves redesigning care homes to meet the current needs of older people, and supporting new initiatives for people with dementia within Falkirk Council Housing and Social Work Services.

Maria Parsons has been involved in social work practice, management, training and lecturing for over 20 years. She is currently Senior Policy Officer with the City of

Westminster Council in London and prior to this was head of the Oxford Dementia Centre, which she was instrumental in setting up at Oxford Brookes University.

The PROP group was set up in 1999 by Denise Chaston, partly in response to the distinct needs of younger people with dementia and their carers which were not being served or recognised in the local area and partly in response to personal experience. A carer initially assisted her in this process. A group was formed consisting of both people with dementia and their carers. The group now has a written constitution and manages its own committee meetings. The members organise social events and fundraising activities. Most importantly they provide education, information and support in the local area and further afield. They are also involved in service planning and with Denise have organised stakeholder events. The name People Relying On People comes from the mining community, where the prop is used to support the pit shaft.

Kate Read has been a social worker for over 25 years, including social work management and commissioning. She has a masters degree in social work and also in gerontology. She has been the Executive Director of Dementia Plus for over three years.

Sarah Rhynas is a nurse and a research student in the School of Nursing Studies, University of Edinburgh, where she is pursuing her interest in the nursing care of people who have dementia. She has worked as a staff nurse in acute medicine of the elderly and currently continues to practise part time in acute medicine at the Royal Infirmary of Edinburgh.

Cesar Rodriguez graduated in medicine and surgery in Valencia (Spain) in 1991. He came to the UK in 1994 to train in psychiatry and specialized in psychiatry of old age. He obtained his current substantial post as Consultant in Old Age Psychiatry in Angus in November 2001. His special interest is psychopharmacology in the elderly and he is also interested in mental health law, in particular the Adults with Incapacity (Scotland) Act 2000.

Stephen Wey is an occupational therapist working as part of an Intensive Home Treatment and Rehabilitation Team for people with dementia in the community. They have been doing this for nearly six years. Before working in elderly mental health he had a background working with people with learning disabilities. As well as his occupational therapy degree he has a degree in the behavioural sciences.

Barry Wiggins and **Jenny Fahy** work for the Hammond Care Group, a not-for-profit organization operating aged care services in Sydney and several provincial centres in New South Wales. Barry is a social worker by training, and works as General Manager, Care Services; Jenny is a registered nurse and is the Regional Manager for the Central Coast area north of Sydney. Barry and Jenny worked together to develop and implement this model of care on the NSW Central Coast in 1998/99 and it now operates in five localities, supporting nearly 300 people with dementia.

Subject Index

Added to a page number 'f' denotes a figure and 't' denotes a table.

Author Index